Victorious

Lisa Cooksey-Cannon

Victorious

A Journey Of Hope And Perseverance

Thank God my brain and body started talking to each other within months of my injury. I'm a walking miracle. God could have said other wise and I would still be in a wheelchair, paralyzed from the neck down.

Lisa Cooksey-Cannon

Victorious, A Journey Of Hope And Perseverance

Published in the United States, Mission Possible Press, a Division of Absolute Good Enterprises. AbsoluteGoodEnterprises.com

ISBN: 979-8-9987146-1-0

Printed in the United States of America

Dedication

To all of the service women and men who have served past, present and future.

To anyone who has suffered a traumatic injury and to their caregivers.

Table of Contents

How Lisa 2.0 Came About..1

Everything Changed 15

Letting Go..39

Being Home Is...70

Being Lisa 2.0 74

Mental Health Struggles Affect the Majority Of Us 79

Reflections **85**

A Woman's Point Of View 87

Impact Of My Injury...90

Barry, Lisa's Husband...94

Finding Hope And Perseverance 99

Resources **101**

Journaling.. 103

Ms. Lisa's 7 Life Principles To Provide Peace........ 105

Living My Best Life Play Lists 111

Resources For Veterans 114

A Note From The Publisher................................... 116

Acknowledgements 117

About The Author... 119

Greetings

There were days when my words failed me, and I only had tears to offer. I'm considered an incomplete quadriplegic.

The incomplete is from "not completely severing my spinal cord." My neck is where my spinal cord injury actually took place - it depends on where the injury takes place on how your limbs are affected - from what I understand. My injury affected all four of my limbs. Had I severed my spinal cord, I would have been permanently paralyzed from the neck down. I have a titanium plate between my Cervical Spine C4 and C6 - from the front, it's under the chin, before the collar bone.

I have so many stories of victory and trying to tell each, my fingers can't write fast enough. Just so you know, a lot of the experiences I remember are from my journal, the one I started keeping after I learned to write again. It's amazing how God works.

Before I could imagine it, God knew my journal would turn into a book of stories that would show how He kept me. I'm just the messenger. I pray you are inspired.

Oh, and by the way, I am a walking miracle, and this is *A Journey of Hope and Perseverance*.

Blessings,

Lisa

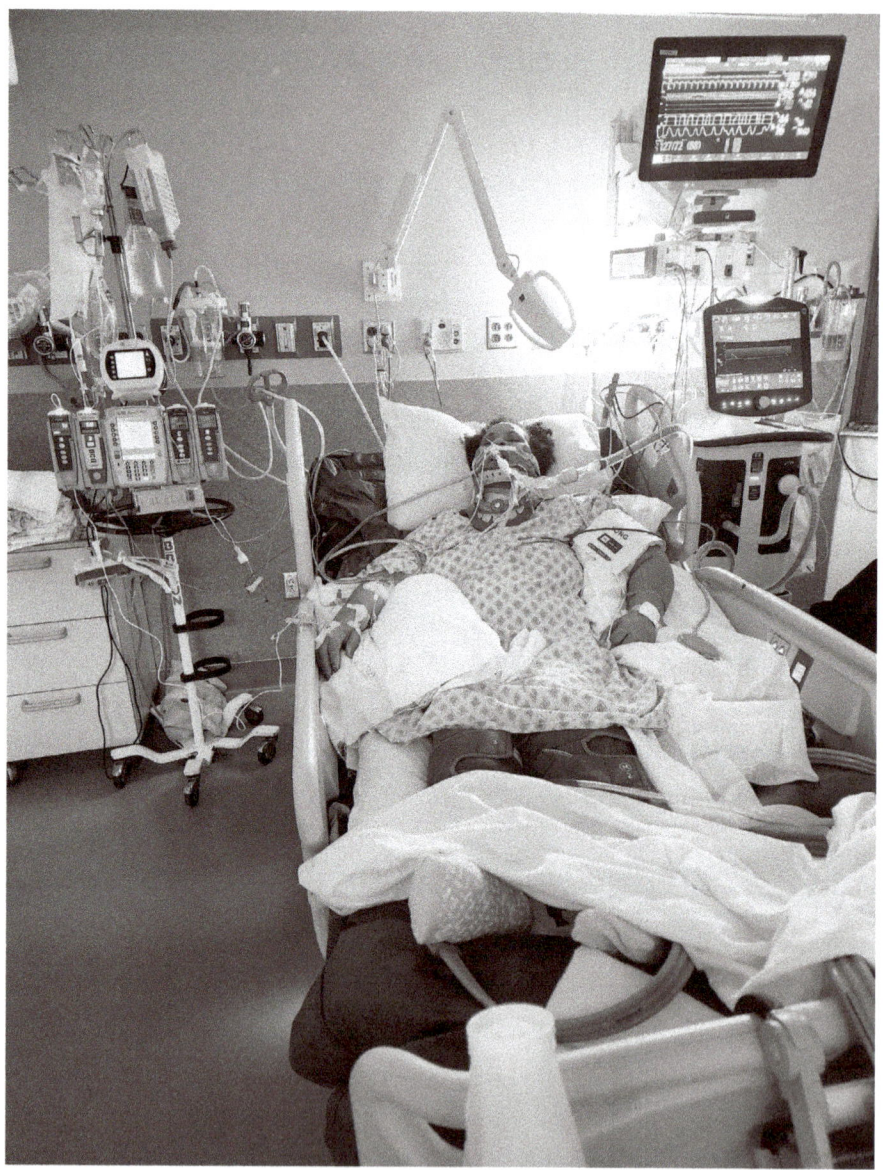

After answered prayers, and the staff saved me.

How Lisa 2.0 Came About

Nobody knows how this "injury" took place.

To this date, I don't remember having a tragic or traumatic event when I felt so much discomfort that I harmed my neck.

My Early Journey

I am Lisa Cooksey-Cannon, a woman seeking God's heart, mother, wife, big sister, aunt, and cousin, veteran, mentor and so on. I grew up in the St. Louis area and graduated from University City High School back in 1983.

After graduation, I attended SEMO (Southeast Missouri State University) in Cape Girardeau, Missouri. I wanted to pursue a degree in Elementary education. I was set on teaching. While I was in school, my mom questioned why I would sign up to "get food stamps in the summer" as a teacher. It sounds funny saying it now, but at that time, it was a real thing. She wanted me to do something different that allowed me to shine a little more. The realities of my choices started sinking in. During my junior year, I became a bit restless. Over the Christmas break, I was working as a manager at a local fast food restaurant. I thought I would give myself a break and not return to school that semester.

Since I was accustomed to living on my own (in the dorms), I figured I needed an apartment in St. Louis instead of staying with my parents. I asked mom to go with me, apartment shopping. She took me to the absolute worst places she could find. The first was above a bar, a freshly painted one bedroom apartment with roaches in every room. I said, "No, let's go to the next one."

We went to the south side of St. Louis. When we pulled up, though there were no chalk lines on the sidewalk, I could've sworn somebody died there. The third one was a rent-a-room with a shared kitchen and bathroom. She made her point. So I decided to stay home with her and my little brother instead of renting an apartment.

I come from a long line of military men; my dad was in the U.S. Air Force, and my grandfather was in the Army. A couple of uncles served in the Army as well. I loved the adventure and the travel they talked about, and that's what drew me to the military.

Being a fast food manager was not for me! It only lasted 3 months and then I quit. I became an aerobics instructor for senior citizens, and enjoyed the exercise and teaching. During that spring, I ran into a friend who had just come back from serving in the Marines for four years. As we were talking, I decided I would try the military.

He started training me on the days I wasn't working, doing push-ups, sit-ups and running, which are major requirements to pass basic training. I loved it. I decided to go visit recruiting stations. I talked to the Marine recruiter first, then I decided to talk it over with my dad. My dad said, "Hell no! Women don't make it in the Marines." My little sister, Teres was headed to the Air Force around the same time, and since I'm a leader and not a copycat, the Air Force was not an option. I decided to join the U.S. Army, and make a career of it.

I headed to Fort Jackson, South Carolina for Basic Training and AIT (Advanced Individual Training). I served on active duty and in the Reserves for approximately 10 years. I started as a 71 Lima, working as a United States Army Administrative Specialist. I was stationed in Germany after AIT, and my sister was stationed in Greece. That gave us the opportunity to travel back and forth and hang out with each other over our first few years. We also took leave and explored many cities throughout the two countries, and also enjoyed France, particularly Paris.

Guess Who Showed Up In Germany? Mr. Barry Cannon.

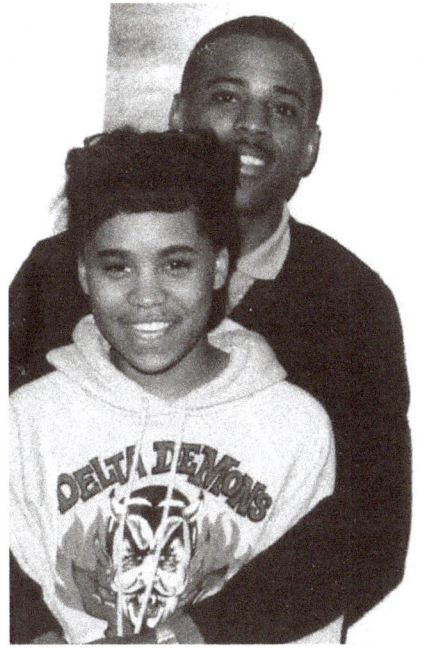

Barry and I in Germany.

I had first met Barry during the summer when I was 14 years old. He was best friends with my mom's younger brother, Gordon. Barry had tagged along with Gordon to my house where I met

3

him and developed an instant crush. He was 15 at the time, and we became a couple. I was not old enough to date, so we "courted." Yes, old school funny. We could sit on my Grandmother's porch and talk on the weekends. He would catch the bus to her house when he had money. When he didn't, he would walk. Believe it or not, we calculated his journey - it was 5.3 miles!

During the week, we could talk on the telephone… yes an actual land line, push button phone with a long white cord so I could sit in a corner for privacy. It was a wonderful summer. Our budding romance ended when Barry left for Atlanta to live with his aunt for his freshman year of high school. I thought of him often, but by the time he came back to St. Louis, I was old enough to date, and was dating a guy with a car. We saw each other occasionally, and through my uncle, he continued to keep tabs on me. All of those long walks helped build his endurance. He enlisted in the Army right after graduating high school. It was my uncle Gordon who was the birdie, tipping Barry off that I was in Germany.

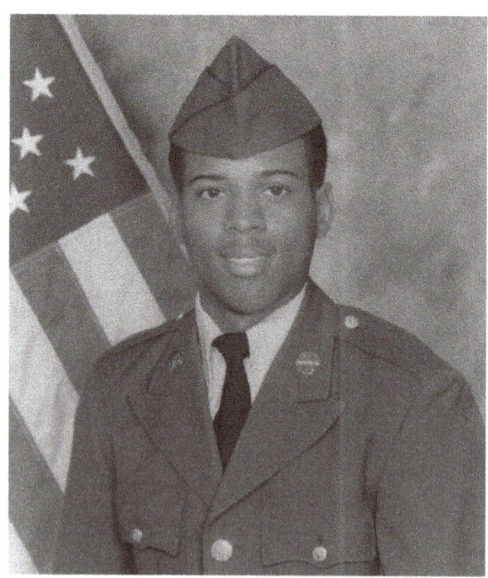

My Love, Barry

Back to Barry in Germany...

We spent the day hanging out and talking. He wasn't ready for a relationship because he had troops he was responsible for. He didn't feel he had time to fulfill his responsibilities and pursue a relationship with me. But he took a professional Army photo of me I'd taken, with him, framed it, and put it on his desk as if I was his girlfriend. We lost touch again.

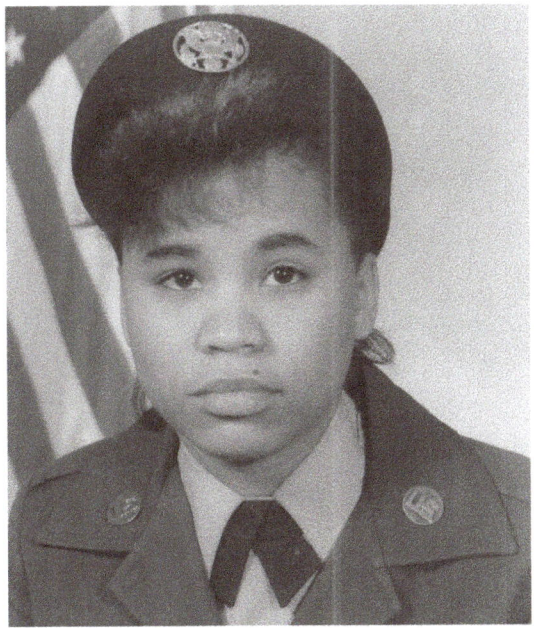

My Official U.S. Army Photo

Life Evolved

I went on to marry an Airman and had my beautiful daughter Amber, who I call my Sweetness. I had served a few years of active duty and joined the Reserves by the time she was born. We lived in Colorado, and I started working for the Department of the Air

Force as an Administrative Assistant. One of the accountants quit without notice, and the CFO of the office asked me if I wanted to train and fill in for her. I agreed. That started my accounting career. It turns out, I was pretty good with numbers.

I was married for 13 years. After divorcing, Amber and I moved to Texas, where I continued my accounting career.

Barry Was Back!

One day, many years later, I received a message from Barry with his name and phone number. I laughed and giggled, remembering how sweet and kind he was, and then I called him. We talked, catching up. He was under the impression I was still married because I hadn't changed my name. Once I told him I was divorced, I think something clicked in his mind and he called me every day, from that day on. Within seven months, we were married. At that time, Barry was retired. He was living in St. Louis after having served 23 years in the U.S. Army. Barry and I have a beautiful love story. So, there you have it, a little bit of tea…

Before My Spinal Cord Injury…

I'm a 'living my best life' kinda girl. That means, hanging out with my husband, attending lots of concerts and musicals, reading my books, journaling, loving on those that love me, having a good time and being thankful that God allows me to experience this good life.

I'm also a 'preparation is key' kinda girl. When I was preparing for work, I would make sure my laundry was done for the week and had my outfits along with jewelry and accessories, and alternate looks ready just in case, all planned out for each week.

I've taken my self-care seriously as well, including regular pamper days at the spa, weekly face masks, and having a dedicated hair washing day. I've also kept up with my yearly exams, followed up with doctors, and I did my best to eat right and exercise at least five days a week. During Covid, I managed to drop some weight, so I was feeling really good about myself. I was even planning to run another half-marathon. I enjoy having goals like this to keep me on task and keep me motivated.

During December of 2023, I Was Living My Best Life!

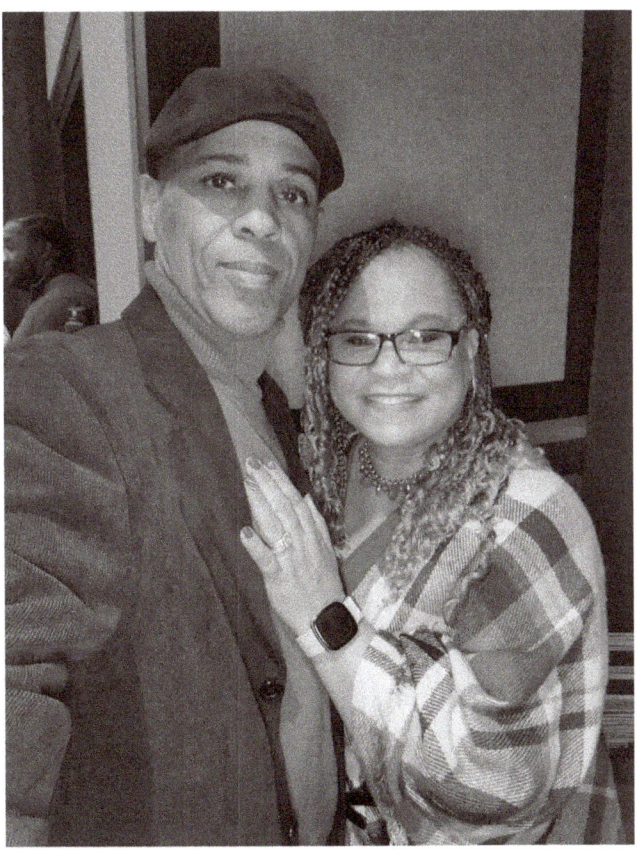

Barry and I, out and about.

Little Did I Know, It Was A Few Weeks Before My Life
Changed Forever

On Saturday, December 2, 2023, I went to see "Renaissance the Movie" featuring Beyoncé. We'd had such a fabulous time at her live concert in August... I love, love, love music, and I felt going to the concert would be a once in a lifetime opportunity. Before going to the concert, I had downloaded her tour playlist and learned each song on the list. And although the concert started an hour late, it was well worth it. I enjoyed every bit of it. It was the best production I had ever seen. So, attending the film, which captured the behind the scenes of that worldwide tour was amazing as well.

Watching the movie in December allowed us to see Beyoncé in her element, wanting to give the people the best concert possible. She was hands on with every detail. Her hustle was strong, and it was a family affair. At each stop on her tour, she was tweaking the production. If she thought it could be better, she would make it so. She had her husband and children with her on tour and showed them behind the scenes rehearsing with her. That was inspiring and touched my heart as a mother. It was so good! My girlfriends and I enjoyed the film so much, and it was a great way to round out the year.

Community service is also very important to me. On Friday, December 8th, I along with members of my Charter Communications Veterans Group, sorted toys to fulfill children's wish lists through the "Toys for Tots" organization. On Saturday, December 16th, we then participated in "Wreaths Across America," at Jefferson Barracks where my dad and my maternal grandparents are buried. Laying wreaths at my loved ones gravesites was such a blessing, and a wonderful way to honor them and their lives. They were each such amazing people, and their memories remind me how much I must do to keep their legacy alive, well and thriving. Participating was heartwarming.

During the middle of December, I vaguely remember waking up to my hands and feet tingling and feeling a little numb. I figured I had just slept wrong and kind of ignored it. It happened again the next day. I mentioned it to My Love. He reminded me I had a doctor's appointment in a couple of weeks, suggesting that I mention it then. I agreed and went about my business.

On Sunday the 17th, some girlfriends and I attended a private showing of "The Color Purple" Movie/Musical. Since I love musicals and music, I really enjoyed Fantasia and the whole cast; they did a really good job.

Oh, and yes, I had a full time job as a Senior Staff Accountant. We worked from home on Mondays and Fridays. On Tuesday the 19th, after my manager came over to chat, I mentioned the numbness and tingling to him. He encouraged me to have it checked out as well.

My Love and I saw Kenny Latimore perform at the City Winery on December 22nd for a wonderful holiday date night.

We enjoyed a family holiday party with my husband's mom and siblings on December 23rd. On Christmas, we took my mother-in-love to the movies; however, she didn't want to stay out too long as she wasn't feeling her best. We didn't think too much of it since it seemed to be "normal stomach issues" for a senior citizen with diabetes and acid reflux.

We had another date night concert at the City Winery on December 26th featuring Mark Harris II. We rode the Ferris Wheel at Union Station on the 29th and then brought in the New Year at home, relaxing on the couch.

January 2024

The first two weeks of the year are extremely important and hectic for accountants. It's the time we must prepare reports of all sorts. It's also kind of an unwritten rule that we don't take off during that season. So, the new year was going pretty well, filled with the normal stress of deadlines, and I was still feeling that tingling and numbness. I tried to ignore it, yet, the feeling had evolved into affecting the functioning of my hands, was lasting longer each time, and had started to become painful. This was the first time my hair had been styled with crochet braids. I started thinking that maybe my braids were too heavy and were causing the numbness, remembering when the stylist had warned me that crochet braids are heavy (with the added hair), even suggesting I may need an aspirin or two when they were being installed.

Wednesday Morning, January 17th

It was a routine visit, during which my doctor asked how I was doing. I mentioned the numbness and tingling, as well as my thoughts about the braids. She said, "Yes, it's possible they may be too heavy." She suggested I take them down as soon as I could. Leaving her office, I felt she confirmed what I was thinking, believing that once I took the braids down, the numbness and tingling would go away.

Friday Evening, January 19th

After work, I start the process of taking down my braids. It's taking a long time, and I'm surprisingly super tired and can barely lift my hands to finish the process. This really concerns me because I had started Thursday night and noticed it was too difficult for me to finish, and just went to bed. Here I was Friday night, struggling with this slow and painful process that had taken over six hours, when it should have been two or three.

Once I finish, I decide to take a shower and wash my hair. I'm in the shower a few minutes and decide I don't have the strength to wash my hair. I am alarmed. I wrap a towel around me, wrap my hair with another towel and barely make it to bed. I fall asleep quickly, completely and utterly exhausted.

Saturday Morning, January 20th

I have to wash my hair, going to bed with wet hair is so not ideal. I drag myself back to the shower and again, I'm too tired to wash my hair. Back to bed I go. My Love is checking on me often. I tell him I'm tired and will get up in a few minutes. I'm in bed the whole day and night.

Sunday Morning, January 21st

I wake up thinking about my chores, going to church and fixing my hair. *What is happening?* I have never experienced this type of pain and exhaustion in my life. I drag myself out of bed to shower and wash my hair. I still have that same towel wrapped around me from Friday. I sit on the commode trying to get enough strength to get into the shower.

I am so weak, I feel as if I'm going to pass out. I can't make it back to bed. I feel myself falling. I don't want to hit my face on the floor. I cup my hands to catch my head as I lean forward. My knees hit the floor as I slide off the commode. I remember turning to lay on my side, there on the bathroom floor. I'm not sure how long I laid there.

The bathroom door was not completely closed, thank God. I slide the door open a bit more, while still on my side. I use my legs to push myself out of the bathroom and into the bedroom...

I have no idea how long I was on the floor. Apparently, I passed out. I opened my eyes and saw My Love. Concerned, he asked why I was on floor. I didn't know. I told him I was too weak to stand. He immediately wanted to call 911. By that time, I wasn't sure about much, but I did know that having strangers see me in a towel was not an option.

"No Sir! Wait a minute, I am not going outta here with all my assets hanging out. PLEASE help me get dressed."

As my husband pulled me up and propped me against the bed frame, I remember thinking, "Why am I so weak?" "My hair is down, why is the numbness and tingling getting worse?" and "I'm too strong to need help getting dressed." As I was in my head, My Love put me in some sweatpants and a T-shirt.

To be on the floor and my husband helping to dress me is a place I never wanted to be. I was embarrassed and would've done anything for My Love not to have to dress me. It was definitely unchartered territory.

911

The fire department arrives first, I'm still out of it. My Love starts to answer questions. The ambulance arrives, followed by the police. My limbs are like *Jello* and my blood pressure is through the roof. The firemen pick me up and put me in a special chair. They carry me downstairs and outside to the ambulance. I'm pretty scared at this point, trying to remain calm and asking God to protect me.

Once I'm on the stretcher in the ambulance, the paramedics take over and start completing a stroke assessment. I'm not having a stroke, which is good. My Love is asking if they can take me over to John Cochran VA Hospital. The paramedics call John Cochran, and I receive approval.

John Cochran VA Hospital Emergency Room

Once I arrive, the doctors are trying to figure out what's causing the numbness, tingling and extreme fatigue. They are running tests, giving me fluids and asking a LOT of questions. I am extremely scared while trying to put on a brave face.

When asked if I'd had an accident or fall recently, I answer, "No."

Shortly thereafter, My Love makes it to the ER (he had driven his vehicle). They ask him the same questions, thinking I may have forgotten something. His answer is the same as mine. I had not experienced any recent trauma.

A few hours later, my test results come back... negative, my blood pressure is back to normal and there is nothing out of the ordinary.

The ER doctor tells me he's going to start my discharge papers, and to follow up with my primary care doctor.

I have some choice words for him, but manage to say, "Excuse me, Sir? I can't walk and my limbs are numb!"

With indifference, the ER doctor instructs me to try and stand.

Okay, let me give it a try.

My Love helps me swing my legs off the bed. I try to stand and my legs are *Jello* again. I'm falling. A big strong male nurse is next to me and catches me mid-fall. He places me back in the bed. Everyone in the room, including the ER doctor can see that though my test results seem normal, my condition is not.

With actual compassion he states, "Let's get you admitted and figure out what's going on." While waiting for a bed to become available, I was too weak to eat. I slept until they transported me up to the 7th floor.

Everything Changed

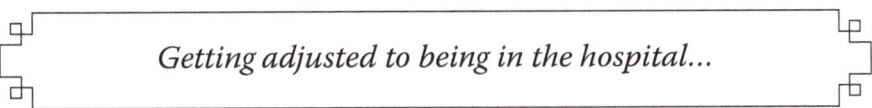

At some point, My Love called my daughter Amber, and my younger sister, Teres. Thinking my situation was nothing major, I remember telling them both not to trouble themselves by coming to St. Louis since I would be home in a few days.

Clearly, other conversations were being had, especially around the seriousness of my then unknown condition. I thank God both of those ladies did not listen to me, and made plans to come immediately.

I finally make it to my room on the 7th floor. It's a two person room. My roommate and I came into the ER at the same time, and I'd heard them speaking to her when I was down there. She had fallen at home and was in need of rehab before she could go home. We hit it off and chatted in between our mutual doctor visits. Being with another female Veteran (*though she was Navy, I didn't hold that against her, lol)*, gave us both a certain amount of comfort.

When they settled me into my room, I was given a walker and told to give my nurse/aide a ring when I needed to go to the ladies room. I pushed the button and she arrived in just under two minutes, which made me hopeful.

She assisted me in walking those few steps to the bathroom. Yes, my legs are a bit wobbly, yet I'm able to take a few steps. I finish tinkling. I try to stand. *Jello* legs again. My aide grabs my shoulders and keeps me from hitting the floor hard. She calls out for help, other nurses/aides come to help me wash my hands and make it back to the bed. Since my knee hit the floor, it was considered a fall. That poor child had tons of paperwork to complete, since a fall is extra.

Now the door has a "fall risk" sign and I have a new wrist band stating the same. I'm exhausted and fall asleep again. The staff put a portable commode by my bed so that I can pivot and take a seat.

A few hours later again, I push the button and my nurse assists me. Literally, I start to crumble in her arms. My knees are on her feet. Thankfully, I didn't make floor contact. Yet, she's stuck and so am I. She can't get me up. I pass out.

When I wake up, there are 10 doctors and nurses looking at me, machines are beeping and my assets are all out for all the world to see.

My nurse is pretty much crying, I scared the crap out of her, and she's a nervous wreck. Once everything calms down, I apologize to her for scaring her. My roommate is shaken as well. Someone calls My Love and informs him of the incident.

Though far past visiting hours, My Love arrives. I can see he is doing his best to be strong and brave for me. Yet, I can finally admit something is drastically wrong with me, based on his composure. After a few hours of watching me go in and out of sleep, Barry and I agree that he'll take my phone back home since I have no strength to hold it.

At this point, I'm told to stay in bed. That further complicated my condition, in my mind. Adjusting to the basics we take for granted, that I could no longer do on my own was extremely difficult, to say the least.

My doctor requested a MRI. The very next morning I'm wheeled down to have the test. I was slid from my bed to the MRI table very gently by the nursing team. The tech asked if I was claustrophobic, to which I replied, "No, I don't think so." He lets me know the machine is loud, the test will take about 20 minutes, and asked me to lay as still as possible. As I enter the machine's tunnel, I ask God to protect me and to please help the doctors' figure out what's going on with me.

Once the test starts the first song that pops into my head is Michael Jackson's "Billie Jean." That seems so weird and random that I decide to change the song in my head. I hear, "Your Spirit" by Tasha Cobbs Leonard featuring Kierra Sheard. They sing:

> *"Not by might, not by power, By Your spirit God, send Your spirit God, Not by might, not by power.*
>
> *By Your spirit God, send Your spirit God..."*

Hearing this calms and gives me energy, joy and peace at the same time. "Your Spirit" is my theme song, reminding me that though I don't have any answers, I trust God through the process.

After completing the MRI successfully, I'm taken back upstairs to the 7th floor and a chaplain comes into my room. God knew what I needed and sent him to pray with me.

The Test Results

Later on that morning, the neurologist comes partially into the room. My Love is in the room with me. We can tell by the look on his face that he's hesitant. He's kinda standing at the door, looking at me and looking at his screen while checking the number on the door to make sure he's in the right place. I don't think he introduced himself, he just started talking out of concern from what he was reading. As he's looking at my MRI results, he states he's never seen someone so young with this much spinal cord damage...

Upon hearing that, My Love and I are looking at each other, now also shaken and concerned. The doctor then he tells me how lucky I am. At this moment, we are panicking because he hasn't yet explained anything.

"You are lucky! Had you moved your head (quickly) to the left or right, you could have severed your spinal cord and been permanently paralyzed from the neck down."

At this point, I'm crying and thanking God for shutting my body down so I would not hurt myself any further... I'm doing the whole ugly cry! *My God, you protected me when I was angry at my body for betraying me. God, You shut my body down to protect me... Thank you Lord.*

After I gather my thoughts, I begin to refocus on the doctor, still standing near the door, but inside the room at this point. He asks if I'd had an accident, taken a fall, or if someone hit me. I answer no, no and no. He's at a loss.

He shows us the MRI results. I had a severely herniated disc that was impinging on my spinal cord. The amount of space between my spinal cord and the bone/disc in my neck was about the width of a fingernail, instead of the width of a finger. This impingement was what was causing the numbness, tingling, severe pain, and my inability to stand or walk; the paralysis.

Discs in the neck should not be pressing against the spinal cord at any point, anatomically speaking. Yet, mine was. It was an extremely rare and serious situation with no plausible explanation.

I don't have words to explain what my husband and I were thinking or feeling in that moment.

By that time, I was having difficulty lifting a fork to feed myself, I couldn't control any movement for the most part, and it was getting worse. The thought that I might actually become "paralyzed" was unfathomable to me.

Snapping me out of my despair and fog the doctor said, "You have two options. You can go home, take your chances and possibly die. Or you can have surgery, with a risk of dying during surgery, but possibly live."

"What?"

"You need surgery immediately to remove the herniated disc and to clean out the bone fragments that are pushing against your spinal cord. We believe this can save you."

All I could do was mumble, "Okay."

The doctor tells us he'll come back in a few moments to have me sign the consent for surgery.

My Love takes my hands and starts to pray for me. We're crying. My roommate is crying. He's praying, and I'm stunned, shocked and afraid to move and of the unknown. I don't quite understand what is happening.

During that prayer, I was telling myself *I know God is a Healer,* and I wanted to take a pill or get a shot. I did not want to be completely paralyzed, nor did I want to have surgery. *How can this be happening? I am not going to freak out!* As my husband's words poured out, I began feeling the presence of the Lord in the room. The Holy Spirit came upon me and gave me the assurance I needed to change my thinking. With my eyes closed, I asked the Lord to help me... my thoughts shifted and I began to pray for a successful surgery.

I signed the consent forms and I was moved to the Intensive Care Unit (ICU) to protect me from any possible further harm until my surgery. I fell asleep somewhere in the stillness of hoping and believing that I would be "okay."

When I woke up, to my surprise, my daughter and sister were sitting next to my bed. They had flown in from California and Alabama to be with me and to support my husband. I am grateful for that time, and that they loved and cared for me enough to be there.

I was in and out of consciousness as the nurses prepped me for surgery. Thankfully, I had a bit of peace, existing in the unknown of my future. I call it faith.

Spinal Cord Surgery

I meet the neurology team. They explain the procedure, and that it should take a few hours. A titanium plate will be placed between my fourth and sixth cervical vertebrae. The C4 controls shoulder movement, breathing and sensation in the neck, shoulders and upper arms. The C5 supports the weight of the head and neck, and kind of acts as a bridge between the C4 and C6. The C6 controls muscles in the wrist and biceps. *No wonder I am having trouble functioning!* Their plan is to "fix" all of this during surgery, after which I'll have to wear a neck brace for the next 12 weeks.

After the neurology team leaves the room, another chaplain comes in and offers to pray with my little family and me just before I'm about to be wheeled into the operating room.

I'm nervous, but I trust God to lead the surgeon's hands and to fix what is broken.

Post Surgery

I asked my husband, my daughter and my sister to fill in the blanks of what I could not recall, so some of the events I'm now speaking about are coming from them.

I wake up after surgery and My Love, daughter and sister are all there. I'm groggy. There are a few tubes along with oxygen, meds and monitors. My neurology team tells me there were no complications during the surgery. They asked me to lift my hand off the bed. All I could do was wiggle my fingers and move my feet a little. Though my family and I didn't know it at the time, that was not good news. If the procedure had been successful I would have been able to perform those simple tasks. Without missing a beat, and hoping to keep me encouraged, the surgeons said they would come back tomorrow and check my progress after the swelling goes down.

In the meantime, my family is there keeping me company. We're watching TV and chatting. My spirits are up, but I can see the worry on the faces of my loved ones. Everyone is used to me being the person who provides the comfort and guidance. My heart aches for them. *I gotta get myself back to normal. I need to do it now.*

Looking back on it, we were all doing our best to remain strong, but we didn't necessarily feel strong. In my mind and heart, I'm thanking God for seeing me through the surgery. I'm hopeful and praying for a swift recovery. I'm ready to be 'back to normal' to take care of them, rather than the reverse.

The next day the neuro team comes in to check my progress. There is no improvement. My doctors are once again at a loss - I should have been able to move. I could not move. The neuro team decides that I need a second surgery. They want to go back in and clean out more of the bone pressing on my spinal cord. To do that, they will have to move my esophagus to reach the area. This news is devastating. I'm still out of it. My Love has to sign all of the paperwork in my place because at this point I'm not able to lift my hands, hold a pen, feed myself or anything. I am completely paralyzed.

A Veteran's Passing

While in the ICU, one of the older veterans died. Prior to his passing, he had coded, but they were able to resuscitate him. That code blue had jarred and concerned me. Though I had not met him, I was sympathetic. I started asking about him, and how he was doing. The staff couldn't tell me much. So, since I knew he was not doing well, I prayed for him and his family daily.

Every day before he passed, I saw several family members come to say their good-byes. During his final days and transition, the staff were so caring and provided for the family's every need. It was very touching. I could feel the love. When he passed, the staff allowed his family to stay with him for a little while. I could tell from the tears he was one of the patriarchs of their family.

As they wheeled him out of his room, over the loud speaker came instructions for all who could to stand at attention or place our hands over our hearts out of respect. It was just a beautiful moment to honor him. To this day I pray for his family and ask God to continue to give them strength and guidance. We've all lost someone we've loved. When I lost my grandparents and my parents, it was difficult, to say the least. Through the grieving process, I've learned to lean into those feelings and allow God to help me heal.

Surgery #2

My family prayed with me before the second surgery. This surgery also took a few hours. Afterwards, I was back to ICU to recover, again. The next day, they tested me to see if there were any improvements. I was able to lift my hands and feet off of the bed! Hallelujah!

My family and I were excited for the progress. However, we did not know that the surgeons expected me to also be able to move and flex my elbows and legs. I was not able, though I was willing.

My husband overheard the doctors talking about me in the hallway, "I've done all I can and I'm unsure of why she can't move."

Nobody mentioned that to me.

At first, I was being fed through my feeding tube, as my throat was still too swollen to properly swallow any food. So for several weeks, I lived on coffee, apple sauce and pudding. That too, was an adjustment, and I lost about 10 pounds during my stay.

I believe the LORD used my situation to show us all how faith and belief in Him works. Yes, the surgeon's hands were directed by God to do what they could medically, but He was destined to get the glory. Just when they thought I would be in a wheelchair forever, God waited a few extra days to move my arms and legs. Every day while visiting, my daughter helps me exercise, rubbing and lotioning my limbs. They wanted me up and moving to lessen the atrophy in my muscles. My progress seemed a bit slow, yet, I was optimistic and surrounded by love.

I wanted to start rehab as soon as possible; however, I had to be off of the oxygen and feeding tube before that could happen. The goal was to transfer to Jefferson Barracks for rehabilitation. However, they had a limited number of beds. My JC neuro team communicated to JB that I was a fighter and that they were my best chance for recovery. JB agreed to hold a bed for me, but I needed to get there as soon as possible.

The Occupational Therapy & Physical Therapy reps came down to show me different exercises to do in preparation of my transfer to JB. Each day I'm getting stronger, but I cannot seem to catch my breath, my throat is still swollen and it's hard to swallow. A few more days go by, I'm coughing a lot and having a hard time breathing. I have been coughing up phlegm and my chest is sore. OT and PT visit every day and show my husband, daughter and sister what to do to help me get stronger. I know I'm feeling better because I ask someone to brush my teeth for me - something I hadn't thought about in weeks.

My daughter is ALL in. She's researching what rehab is going to look like for me, and letting me know it's going to be tough. She tells me to concentrate on small victories daily. When she said that, it sounded good and felt right. Concentrating on small victories daily became my victory motto. It is a phrase I speak every morning after my prayers.

Upon further examination, the doctors realize I have pneumonia a few days after my second surgery. I'm choking on everything, including clear liquids though the ENT team teaches me exercises to help me swallow without choking, nothing's helping.

I am telling myself I shall push through and continue to get better.

Mid-morning, Barry, Amber and I are watching something on daytime TV while my sister was off running errands. Then it all fades to black...

Barry later told me what happened. All of a sudden I was quiet. He turned to me and saw my eyes roll toward the back of my head as my blood pressure was steadily rising.

When the BP monitor approached 260, the ICU doctor on duty rushed into the room yelling my name, "Ms. Cooksey! Are you ok, Ms. Cooksey? Can you hear me?"

My blood pressure is over 280. A nurse runs in, "She's going to have a..." and stops midsentence before saying the word stroke, when she sees my love and daughter in the room. I am unresponsive. My family is escorted out of the room as the team was rushing in.

In the waiting room, Amber asked My Love if she could pray. "Of course."

She named every doctor, nurse, tech, every person she could think off that had a hand in my care. The prayer was so mighty and powerful that My Love was sure God and all the angels heard her prayer. When they said, "Amen," everyone seated in the waiting room said Amen as well. Shocked at what they heard, they looked around, not having realize anyone else was in the waiting room.

During and after that prayer, there were several codes called on my room, including code blue. My husband and daughter were not sure if I had died.

Lord have mercy.

From what I'm told, they worked on me for about an hour; finally I was stable.

Before going back into my room, the doctor told Barry and Amber I had been intubated. Since my daughter had been an Army medic, she knew what that meant. The doctor explained to My Love that a tube was breathing for me, and warned them of all of the tubes, hoses and such that they would see. He also reminded them that I was alive and that I was sedated. I could possibly hear them, but would not be able to respond.

They came into my hospital room and both broke down seeing me with the ventilator tube, my oxygen tube, my med tubes, my vitals tube and a feeding tube, with my blood pressure at 218... still dangerously high. Through their fear and tears, they begin talking and ministering to me with words of encouragement and prayers.

We were spent. A few hours later, they headed home after what had been a traumatic day for all of us. Later, they both admitted they had eaten quickly and fell asleep before 5pm, exhausted.

The fact that my daughter and sister left their families to come see about me and to support my husband, truly shows their loving and giving spirits, women who love God and me enough to drop everything and see about me. I remain so very grateful for every moment they were here to support me and My Love.

My heart still aches for this stressful part of my journey. Thinking of what my family witnessed and experienced, makes me sad, because I would never want this for them.

Barry and Amber visited the next morning and evening - no change. I was still resting.

I have no outside memory of those 48 hours. I had no cares in this world. I just know God was healing my body during that extreme time of rest.

During the time I was unconscious, I do remember hearing music, like an orchestra, with horns and violins sounding each time I took a breath.

God said to me, "Go back to sleep, you need to rest."

Was I semi-conscious? I don't know. I heard Him, my LORD speaking to me, healing me. I closed my eyes and continued resting.

***

The next morning, when I opened my eyes, Barry, Amber and my doctors were there smiling. The doctor said with confidence, "You're a fighter."

I believed him.

"We're going to take that tube out. I need you to take a deep breath."

The tube was out. I was good.

One of the ICU nurses said, "We don't have many patients who come off the ventilator in 48 hours. We knew you were strong, but jeezz! You have everyone in the ICU smiling today!"

I had NO idea what was happening. I realized it was a good thing.

My Love told me a short while later that my blood pressure spiked again. The numbers were ticking up steadily and quickly like when you're filling up your tank at the gas station. I was out again.

This time they administered new blood pressure medication quickly. I did not code. Evidently, I just needed to rest. Overnight, my blood pressure was back to a safe number - thankfully.

That next morning when I woke up, I felt better, refreshed. Finally, I was starting to recover, according to the doctors.

God allowed me to make it through the storm.

About three weeks after being admitted to the hospital, my family was visiting. I casually used my right hand and scratched my nose!

We laughed, and told the staff to come in so I could do it again!

I know it sounds silly, but to a person that's been paralyzed for weeks THIS IS A BIG DEAL and a great turning point in my physical recovery. Yes, it was another small victory!

Side Effects

My brain is struggling with nightmares, insomnia and hallucinations which started after my first surgery and persisted nightly. I was seeing rats, birds and some stranger standing over me. It was horrific. I prayed them away every night, yet my mind, my mental state, and my well-being were fragile. This was so abnormal for me that I finally mentioned it to the doctor. He said it was likely a side-effect of one of my necessary medications. That was tough to hear, but I needed sleep.

He explained that I needed that medication for my recovery, but that he would give me another medicine to hopefully stop those side effects. I took it. The hallucinations stopped after a couple of days although I still suffer with nightmares and insomnia, unfortunately.

Issues Of Life

During my time in ICU, My Love is taking care of all of the household responsibilities. Fortunately, the accountant in me had already paid the bills in advance, as my normal habit. However, there were many things Barry was juggling including household chore busywork, my FMLA paperwork, appointments for himself, driving my daughter and sister around and dropping them off to visit with me. During that time, he was also trying to figure out what was happening with his Mom and her health, as she was declining, unbeknownst to the rest of us.

He was monitoring my calls and text messages and trying to protect my privacy by requesting no visitors and no phone calls. He made that decision because we were so uncertain about my health; we only wanted good energy and healing thoughts. It was a lot to handle. He did request that our home church pray for me. My Love was drained mentally, physically and spiritually. Yet, he showed strength and resilience whenever he was in my presence. I thank God for keeping him supplied with perseverance and guidance.

Back In ICU

Each day a tube was removed, thankfully. I wanted to start rehabilitation ASAP. Rehab would not accept me unless I was stable and ready to work. After nearly a month in ICU, I was cleared to start rehab. That night, before leaving the ICU, my daughter left a note on the whiteboard in my room, thanking everyone for taking such good care of me and answering all of our questions.

The day before leaving the hospital, I spent one day on the Spinal Cord Injury floor at John Cochran. The nurses took excellent care of me and explained the rehab process in detail. I remember listening to them and thinking about this next phase of my process. They told me "Rehab is a BEAST! It's hard, it's uncomfortable, and there are so many unknowns."

So many things were on my mind. I needed to rest, but I couldn't sleep. I could not forget what the surgeons had told me - there was still a spot on my lower spine that could possibly require surgery. We would know in a few weeks, following another MRI.

Whew! My head was spinning. *Jesus, I cannot go through this again!*

I prayed for more small victories. I still had no ability to hold anything in my hands. That meant I could not read the Bible on my phone or in the book itself. That night I lay in bed and recalled Matthew 9:20.

> *Just then a woman who had been subject to bleeding for twelve years came up behind Him and touched the edge of his cloak. She said to herself, "If I only touch his cloak, I will be healed."*

I just needed to touch the hem of His garment.

I was reciting that scripture daily. I prayed for continued heal-ing, courage, strength, patience, my family and the ability to walk again. At some point, during this intimate time with God, I fell asleep in peace, grateful and hopeful.

The fact that My Love had to see me like that, just helpless, and they had to live through it still makes me cry. Not knowing if I was going to make it. It just breaks my heart that they had to see me like that day in and day out. I guess I'm so used to being the one that picks everybody up and giving them what they need. I couldn't give them what they needed (she is crying!). You never want the people whom you love to hurt like that.

I feel guilty and responsible for their pain. I've felt like my body betrayed me, and that's one of the times I felt like it betrayed me, but looking at it, I immediately knew it was God allowing me to rest and heal. But I was still mad.

And that man, I love him. Since being that little girl, I've always loved him. And I never want him to hurt like that. That's how I knew, when I woke up and saw them smiling, I knew I had to fight. I knew something good had to come out of it. But the pain I saw in their faces let me know that whatever had happened was not good. No one told me what had happened until months later. And I think at some point - I think my sister is still too fragile, too afraid to talk about it.

One day when I was in the hospital my sister said, "I need you to get better because trying to be the big sister sucks."

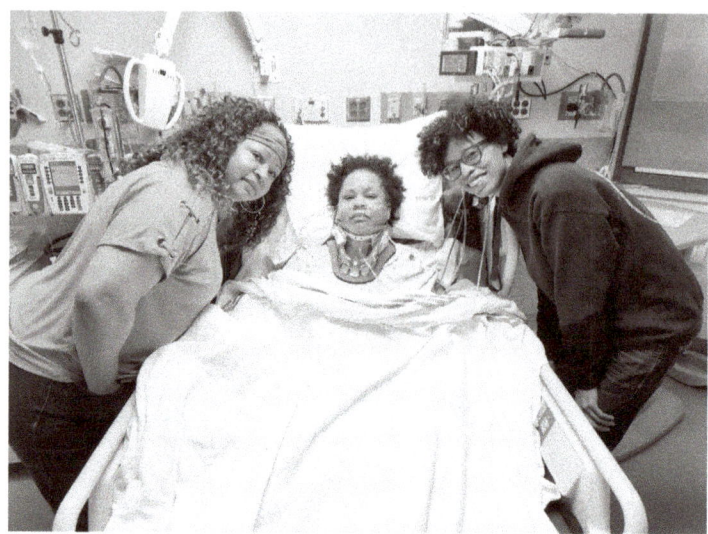

My sister, Teres, Me and my daughter, Amber.

Off To Rehab At Jefferson Barracks

I was transported to Jefferson Barracks Spinal Cord Unit, Building 52 by way of ambulance in mid-February 2024. Though it was a long and bumpy ride, I was alive! I was outside for the first time in nearly a month! The sun was shining! It was a good day!

I was rolled into my room. Many of the nurses and staff came in to introduce themselves; so many faces and names. One nurse in particular, Mo, whispered in my ear "We've got you queen." I immediately felt a peace within my spirit. When she squeezed my hand, I knew someone was going to help me through this process.

The intake nurse came in and got straight to work... A million questions! Whew child, it took some time!

The best part of the intake process was the opportunity to "pick my team." They honored my request to have all females aid me in my recovery as I wanted ladies around to care for me. I was so grateful. Though I'm jumping ahead a bit, I quickly realized most of the nurses and techs were beautiful women who cared for me as if I was a sister, aunt or daughter. My team consisted of doctors, nurses, occupational therapists, physical therapists, a dietician, a psychologist, and a social worker.

After intake was completed, Amy from PT came in to access the situation. I asked if I could sit up in a chair since being immobile for such a long time is hard on a person mentally and physically. I was told no. I had to stay in bed until the doctors reevaluated me, and it was safe. The saving grace is I will able to sit in a wheelchair and be semi-mobile as a result.

Amy wanted me to be fitted for a wheelchair and start therapy the next day. Amy kind of laughed as she asked, "How tall are you?"

I responded with a mighty loud voice, very confidently, "Five feet even."

She smiled, I knew she was thinking this short lady is very happy with her whole 5 feet even self... Amy knew I was on the shorter side because the bed was swallowing me up.

Those beds are for grown men that I am NOT. It started on the first day. Each time the staff came into my room they would prop me back up in my bed because I was sliding down. And I was supposed to be rested on the sling to make it easier for them to move me when needed.

It was funny at times, me sliding. Since I could not move, I stayed in that position until someone came in and pulled me back up onto the pillows. Once pillows were used to prop up my feet, I did not slide as much. The sling is used to move me from my bed to the wheelchair. They had to find and order a smaller hoist for me, as I almost fell out a few times, again it's made for big, grown men.

The spinal cord unit was accustomed to having large and extra-large hoists for patients.

In addition to fulfilling many other needs, RaShonda, my social worker, was the glue to keep everyone, including all team members, my family and friends informed of my progress through weekly calls and meetings. Having a friendly, hardworking and kind social worker who was so vested in my recovery made the process seamless. The way she managed my case worked well, and provided a whole health approach.

Also, I was not alone, there was another female veteran in rehab, named Ginger. They had not had two female veterans in the unit at the same time in forever. We come with a whole new set of challenges. I'll mention a few as we continue this journey.

Getting To Physical Therapy (PT) Is A Process

It took a few days to start therapy because they were looking for a smaller wheelchair for me. Once they found one, they used the sling and hoist with hooks to lift me from my bed to the wheelchair. That first time was when we all noticed I was too tiny for the apparatus, but we made it work.

My first few therapy visits were focused on testing. They helped me exercise because I couldn't move on my own. They would put something in my hand and roll it around to see if I could feel it. Then I tell them what I think the object is.

At this point, I am still unable to use any part of my body below my neck. I can't really move my neck because I am wearing a neck brace. The surgery gave me the ability to move; however, it would take physical and occupational therapy to give me the practice of movement throughout my body to relearn everything.

Gradually, when they position my arm properly, I can move my right pointer finger on my own. Since that finger is now working, I am able to guide the wheelchair on my own. I am overjoyed to be out of bed and guiding the wheelchair myself. Even though the chair is set to turtle mode - the slowest it can actually go, slower than walking at a normal pace - it is a victory to me!

There were several days at PT/OT when whomever escorted me to therapy would steer my wheelchair back to my room as I was too exhausted to put my hand on the arm rest and guide with my finger. Plus, in the beginning trying to get the hang of guiding, getting the right speed and turning the wheelchair to the left or right was a challenging. Plus, I had to wear these big blue boots and compression socks. The blue boots were to protect my feet just in case I ran into a wall or cut a corner too close. It's easy for a paralyzed person to break a foot or toe and not even know it because you have no feeling in your feet.

I know, let that sink in. #ButGod

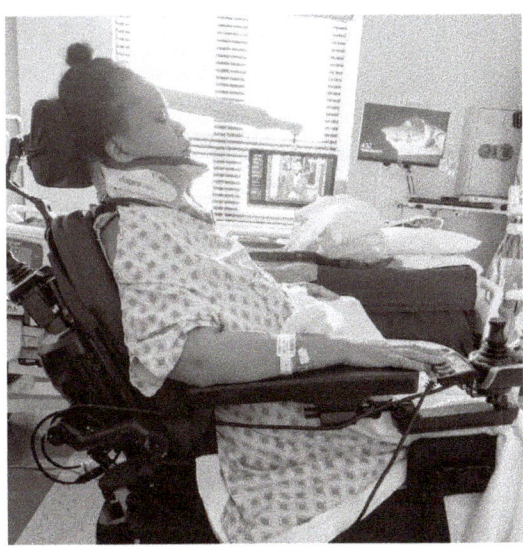

Navigating the wheelchair.

God and Provision

Shortly after arriving, Pastor Cynthia, the JB Chaplain, introduced herself and asked if I was interested in attending church. Yes! I was excited. I had to get prepared for my first Sunday. I had been wearing huge men's pajamas for my first days in PT and OT. I guess I hadn't thought too much about clothes until thinking about church. Though I would have enjoyed being in service with my husband, I wanted him to rest, so I asked him to bring some clothes and other personal items for service and for my rehab stay in general.

On my first Sunday at church, one of the techs escorted me down to church. We parked my wheelchair next to a pew. I thought I would see the other Veterans from the spinal cord unit. Nope, just me and one other guy. Oh well, their loss. Though, I could not hold the worship service program, my tech turned the pages for me so I could follow along. My first service was just what I needed. I needed God's Word to keep me going. Coming to the realization that I may have to spend the rest of my life in this wheelchair was very scary. As the Chaplain was preaching, all I could do was cry. My throat was still raw. My words were very scratchy and low. So crying was my way of worshipping. During that service, I let go of some of my pain as well. I earnestly thanked God for His grace and mercy... and for my life... no matter how this hospital stay would turn out.

I invited Ginger to service the next week, and she joined us. From that point on, we made it a thing.

***

I had many other challenges and adventures. You have to build up your endurance for PT and OT. I would sweat as though I had run a marathon and would fall asleep after every session.

Being in a wheelchair you have to release the pressure on your spine. So you go into a tilt - meaning, using the button on the wheelchair which tilts you back to release the pressure. You are supposed to tilt every 30 mins or so, and stay in this tilted position for about five minutes.

One day after lunch, I needed to tilt so I tilted the wheelchair back, and fell asleep. My tech Valerie had taken away my tray and stated she would be back in 30 mins to escort me back to therapy. She said she walked by and saw I was tilted, no biggie. She walked by my room again 15 minutes later and I was still tilted, still no biggie. She came by again and rushed in the room calling my name. She did not realize I had fallen asleep and was worried because I was in tilt mode for a good 45 minutes. When she woke me up I was fine, just tired.

My approach to therapy was being open and agreeable to whatever task, exercise or process was asked or expected of me. I would never tell them no, and no matter how grueling or difficult things would get, I would always try my best. I applied this approach to any and every task given.

Focus and rest were so important during this time, that I asked My Love to only come over to visit every other day, instead of daily, after 6 pm and no other visitors during the week if possible. There was nothing cute about me falling out and snoring loudly in front of my husband or anyone else. A girl needed her beauty rest.

That's how exhausting therapy was for me.

Since the body needs time to recover and rest, I did not have PT or OT on the weekends. The strenuous exercises were reserved for the weekdays, thankfully. On the weekends, I used a hand grip along with bands to move my fingers, forearms and do curls. By this time, my daughter and sister had returned to their homes, keeping in touch through the weekly meetings and when My Love got them on the phone during his visits. I was busy with other family and friends visiting, which was great!

I needed to see them, and I drew inspiration from everyone's encouraging words, thoughtful gestures and updates from the outside world.

Letting Go

Growing up, my dad made sure I was confident and capable of maintaining my own being. He saw how tiny I was in stature and knew I would be a target for bullies. Therefore, he wanted to make sure I could stand on my own, and he did a great job. Although I needed that affirmation to keep me confident in my youth, there's a softer side I needed to show as well, especially as a young woman. Sometimes I buried the girlie part of me when I needed it to show the most.

Releasing Control

It's really tough when you're used to doing things a certain way. All of that goes out of the window when you're paralyzed. Allowing others to take care of you, the way you take care of everyone else, and not letting your ego get in the way of asking for or accepting help is essential to recovery and to day to day quality of life, no matter your physical or mental state.

Especially as a veteran, I got accustomed to figuring things out and being tough despite any circumstance - which is excellent for survival - but not always the best way when it comes to maintaining relationships with others. Sometimes we want to be so independent that we'll suffer through things, and 'do it ourselves' when it would be better to ask for help. When we are willing to release control, and let go, it can make it easier for us and everyone involved, especially when they are dedicated and committed to supporting us. I'm saying this because it's still difficult, though I've been Victorious through so much, to allow others to "help me." *The lesson?* When I trust those who have proven time and time again that I can count on them, the journey is much easier to travel - together.

During my recovery and rehabilitation at Jefferson Barracks (JB), I met with my doctors for daily check-ins to make sure I was feeling okay, my meds were working the way they should and to address any concerns my family or I have. My nurses and techs were with me every step of the way, with me all day, supporting me through the entire process. At first, in my mind, it was difficult to allow them to do those very personal things for me, however, I really had no choice, since I could not move my body and do them for myself. I almost hate to admit it, but I think it took something this big and serious to allow me to let go enough, and humble myself enough, to allow the help, care and support I needed and deserved.

Karaoke And Friendship

Once I arrived at JB I had a swallow team who visited me every few days and provided exercises to strengthen my throat muscles. This whole team approach worked so well. Each member of my team made sure everyone on the team was immediately made aware of any concerns, adjustments and accomplishments.

I attended a Karaoke event in the gym shortly after that. I was wheeled in by one of the techs, and was placed next to Ginger, the other female veteran with the spinal cord injury who struggled to fit the apparatus they had available for us. My friendship with Ginger inspired me daily. When I met her, she was able to use the wheelchair and was also able to walk with the use of an upright walker. Ginger has the best smile ever. We quickly became friends, God knew I needed her. Only someone that's going through what you're going through will truly understand your struggle. The Karaoke experience was almost surreal. Being in that big space, surrounded by other veterans in various conditions made me glad to see them. I felt like I had found my tribe. Before that, I had felt so isolated.

I noticed a couple of guys that used a mouth-piece to guide their wheelchairs because they were completely and permanently paralyzed. All they would ever be able to do would be to guide themselves that way, nothing else. Seeing them was humbling. I felt so bad for them, and at the same time, I just felt that somehow, my outcome would be different. Being with my fellow vets put me at ease. I was there being obedient, believing that God's will for me, whatever it would be, would be okay, no matter the ultimate outcome.

There were snacks and plenty of people taking turns singing. Although I could not eat or drink any of the refreshments, at that point I was able to sing very softly. That experience is a treasured memory, and I enjoyed singing some of my favorite songs. Though my belly wasn't fed, my soul was.

Personal Care Matters

I've said this before, it's takes a special person to brush your teeth for you, wash your face, help you dress and wipe your bottom with such care and grace. I was surrounded by several special persons doing this for me.

My techs learned how much I enjoyed music and created a wonderful environment. Each day for lunch, my Smooth Jazz was playing and my room smelled wonderful. They made my home away from home neat, clean and welcoming. Those little things made a big impact.

Without me knowing or even thinking about it, my neuro surgeon had operated on my neck very specifically, keeping the location in mind to minimize the scar by placing it in the crease of my neck. This was an intentional gesture which I truly appreciate. It's also reflective of other acts of kindness I experienced during my journey.

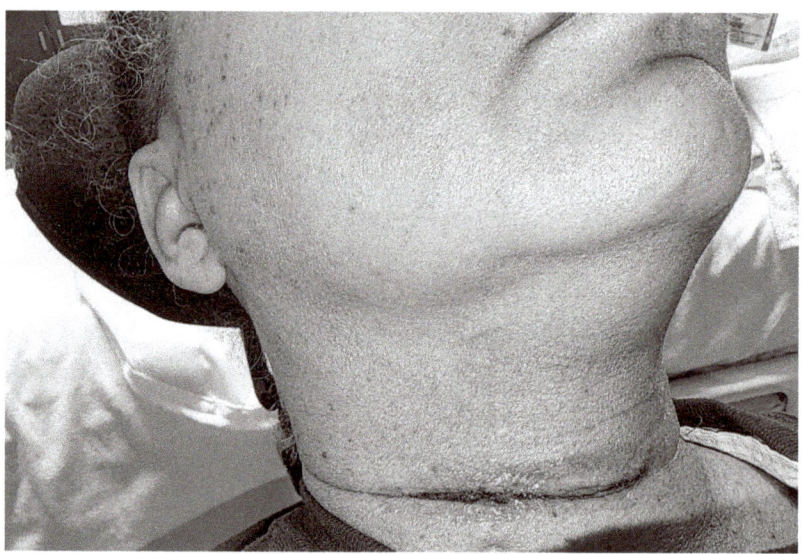

Exceptional scar placement.

After about two weeks in JB, one of the neuro nurses came in to examine my neck. He checked the scar, and it looked great to him (I still had not seen it at that point). He also checked my neck, and overall, it was healing well. He cleared me to take off my neck brace to eat. The neck brace was designed to keep me confined and safe - rendering me unable to move, to protect me. With it off during meals, I finally felt moments of freedom - and that I was healing! This did so much for my mind and my mindset, I remember feeling what it was like being *Victorious*, one step at a time.

Without me asking, friends had brought me head scarves and Nurse Brenda had even stopped at the beauty supply store on her way in one day and brought me some hair products. She had even brought me a bonnet. This helped a bit, but my hair was in such bad shape, and was so matted, I actually thought maybe I should cut it off and start again.

I'll never forget that Saturday when Lynn, one of my precious techs, took all day to wash my hair and braid it up for me. At that point, my hair had not been touched since I had begun taking down those braids when I lost consciousness in my bathroom that Sunday morning a month and a half prior.

She took the time to gently detangle my hair as much as she could before washing and conditioning it in the shower, then detangling again. She was so careful and gentle not to strain my neck or get my bandage wet, while also getting through that nest which had bothered me so. During the process, I was scared and relieved at the same time. By Saturday night, I was so exhausted, I didn't have company that night, I just fell asleep, feeling more like myself, while claiming another small victory.

Occupational Therapy Is Hard And Necessary Work

OT works your upper body, arms, hands, fine motor skills, etc. The goal was to help me learn how to bathe, clothe myself, and to write and feed myself again, among other critical things.

There were a few nights I had a big attitude. I was tired and in pain physically and mentally. I just wanted to be in bed and rest, peacefully. Whenever I had to wait to be put in bed, or for one of the techs to feed me, I checked myself and my attitude. I got over it quickly and used the time to get in a few more hand/arm exercises, once I was strong enough to do them. *Use your time wisely,* I told myself.

It's also a challenge to complete leg lifts when you have no feeling in your extremities. I was determined to work hard whether I could feel the movement or not. I knew the harder I worked, the harder the OT and PT team would work with me.

Every day I pushed a little harder. During rehab, I also attended virtual educational classes. Those classes are designed to make you aware of what's happening with your body. That's important because each time therapy started, they reminded us that every spinal cord injury is different. Meaning, they would work with me at my own pace. I took that to mean to keep my eyes focused on God.

Food

During rehab my diet changed from coffee, apple sauce and pudding to the "Minced and Moist Menu." Everything is minced and strained like baby food. It's so disgusting. *I'm shaking my head even thinking about it.*

I could only eat minced and moist because at the time I had a disorder called dysphagia. As I progressed, the swallow team would visit and watch me eat. One bite, chew 4,287 times... lol. Swallow, take a drink of water, then take another bite. I had to take my time so that I was not choking on my food nor was it going down the wrong pipe, which happened a lot in the beginning.

With each meal, the tech who brought in my food trays would laugh as we read the menu and then smelled the food to try and figure out which "minced" or "moist" dish it was.

One day for breakfast, I had eggs, sausage and pancakes. We know eggs are yellow. But the pancakes and sausage were almost the same color. How do you mince a pancake? So I did a taste test and I could taste a little spicy in the darker brown in the minced combo and decided that was the sausage. The lighter brown mystery turned out to be the pancake, which did have a little bit of syrup to sweeten it up. That syrup was like having desert. Just know, I will never eat anything minced such as zucchini (which was the absolute worst), carrots or peas again. It was disgusting. There was not enough salt, pepper, ketchup, butter or anything else that would make those vegetables good. Just in case you're wondering there is NOTHING good about minced and moist. As if my description was not enough, I need you to understand how difficult eating was during my journey.

Stages Of Minced And Moist

❖ Level 1 is basically water or juice
❖ Level 2 slightly thick liquids like nectar
❖ Level 3 mildly thicker liquids like honey
❖ Level 4 pudding
❖ Level 5 is minced and moist like mashed potatoes with gravy or blended chicken with sauce. (Yes, solid foods were blended in a blender or finely chopped with some type of sauce - moistness). Yuck!!!
❖ Level 6 soft and bite sized scrambled egg
❖ Level 7 a regular diet

Yes, eating was a chore; however I had to get down as much "food" as I could. I needed my strength to make it through PT/OT every day.

Since I was unable to feed myself, my tech would feed me. Then I would listen to Smooth Jazz or Gospel music until it was time to head back to therapy for a second time daily. I was exhausted so much of the time that the music helped me relax and rest after consuming my "scrumptious" lunches.

Each week, my family and I met with my entire team. Each week, those teams would lay out what I accomplished that week and set goals for the next week. I thank God for His consistent provision. During therapy they will tell you not to be alarmed if you stay stagnant or do not make any progress; it's a part of the process. I'm so thankful. Each week I progressed. I was not stagnant and did not take any steps backwards.

Moving My Upper Body And Feeding Myself Again

Occupational therapy provided exercises to strengthen my upper body. A day in OT would consist of arm exercises, pull downs, bicep curls and chest presses, for example. I would also do hand exercises using a ball of clay, pulling the clay apart to find the tiny light bulbs or tiny beads. There was also a large plastic bin filled with rice. I was to sort through the rice and find as many objects as I could in a specified time, with my eyes closed, and using both hands. My left side has always been weaker so I focused on working with it a bit more each time I had OT.

Let me tell you about feeding myself. Around the 3rd week in OT, my occupational therapist Kim said on a Friday afternoon, "I think you have gained enough strength in your hands to feed yourself. You should try it tonight."

I had begun to regain feeling in my hands and arms though they were still very numb and tingly. I was able to grasp objects, so I made up my mind I would try it. That evening after my last therapy session of the day, dinner time came, and I told the tech I wanted to try and feed myself... it was an experience!

I have a divided plate, like a kid, to keep my baby food separated, lol. My tech gives me the spoon and I lift it to my mouth. I actually feed myself! Now don't get me wrong, there is more food on my bib than in my stomach, but that is okay!

Experience, expertise and teamwork all played a part during my journey. It's amazing how the staff understands what's needed at any given time. We played a variety of games, with varying levels of complexity. I thought they were fun. And, all the while these activities were strengthening my whole upper body, which I would need to bathe and clothe myself. Eventually, I began to help lift myself up from my wheelchair, to the slide board, to the bed. My favorite game was Snap Circuits, a skill builder game. I loved building those tiny projects, technical projects; its main purpose was using my fine motor skills… Wow.

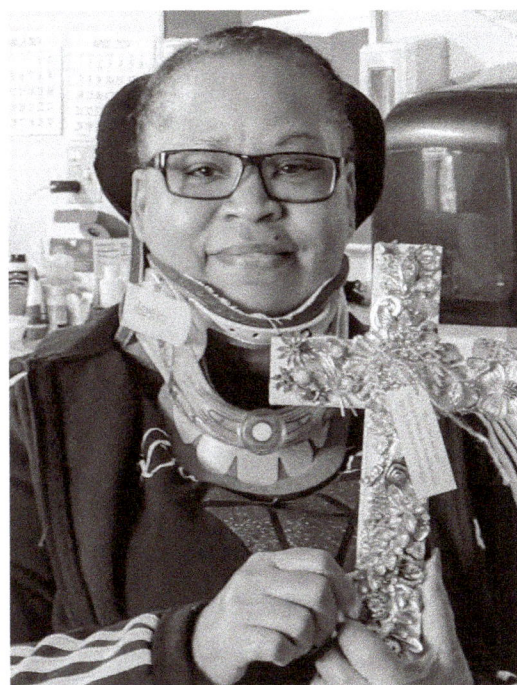

Therapy, customized.

Each time I made progress, the tech immediately put a note in my chart, which everyone on my team could read. From lifting my spoon to victory the first time, to finding little bulbs in clay, each game, activity and exercise strengthened my upper body and my resolve. Everyone was so proud of me, as they continued to encourage me on the easy days and the difficult days. I did have some sleepless nights. I tossed, I turned, and I worried. Yet, when I saw my occupational therapist daily, I gathered my courage to persevere and do my part. And when I felt too weak to continue, I searched my heart, asking for more strength, more willpower, and more perseverance. Daily, I was thanking and acknowledging God for small victories. And daily, he was giving them to me.

My Past Motivated My Present

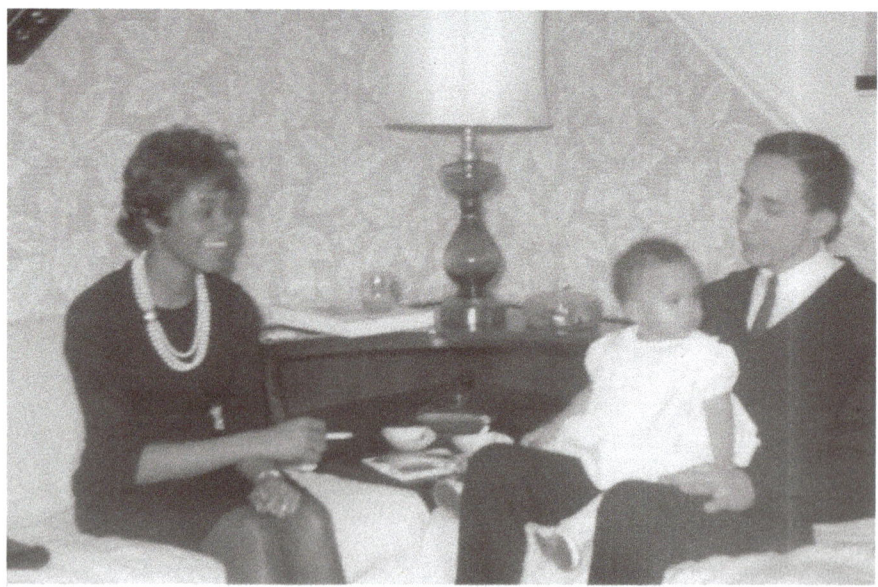

Mom, baby Me, and Dad.

As I mentioned, before my spinal cord injury, I was extremely active, and enjoyed being involved. This started at a young age, with my dad. Being with him was always an adventure.

My mom, Leola, met my dad when she was in high school. They had a good thing going, but she also had the "military bug" and had been recruited into the Air Force. She had planned to be a nurse. My dad, by that time, had already been in the Air Force. After graduating, as she was preparing for service, they discovered me, a bun in the oven. There went her military career. My parents married, had my two other siblings, and then divorced when I was 10 years old.

Although they were divorced, my dad made it clear to us and my mother that she was the love of his life, that he wouldn't marry anyone else, that he would always be there for us and for her; and he was. He took care of all of us.

In her late 20s, Mom started suffering with tremendous pain and was unable to get out of bed for days. Eventually, they diagnosed her condition as being Lupus, so that limited her being able to be active with me and my siblings. Back then, in the 70's they didn't know much about the disease, her flare ups or the other things that were happening with her. So for lack of better words, I would say the doctors kept her 'doped up' because they had no idea how to manage her pain.

During my hospitalization, recovery and rehab, I often thought of both of my parents. I missed them. Loving my mother and admiring her so, I knew I didn't want to be relegated to being in bed the rest of my life. I didn't feel that great about possibly being wheelchair bound either, but it did give me some hope - if I could learn to navigate it.

On the other hand, when thinking of my dad, Theodore, I used our memories as motivation to get up and get active! It was always fun being out with dad. Wherever we went, women would always openly flirt with him in front of my sister and me. I would always wonder why they were acting like that! But, I guess they couldn't help themselves - my daddy was Smokey Robinson fine!

I loved to bowl even though I wasn't very good. My dad loved it as well, and taught me how to do it. He had the best hook ever - whenever he threw the ball, it looked like it was going in the gutter but it never did.

He also taught me to ride a bike, and to swim, roller skate, play pool, play darts and of course, he taught me how to play Spades. He also taught me how to drive in Forest Park. My dad also loved to gamble. He was an experienced Black Jack player. Once I was old enough, he would sometimes take me along to the casino, where I would watch him win.

So on February 29, 2024, I did something I did not know was possible - I went bowling. In the basement of the JB facility was a full bowling alley with maybe 6 lanes or so. I bowled from my wheelchair using an adaptive device I was able to "roll into," which held the bowling ball. There were dots on the ball so I was able to use the dots to bowl, guide the ball a little to the left or right as needed.

Rehab Schedule: **Thursday 2/29/24**

Room #: Last Name:	66-2 *Cooksey- Cannon*
9:00 AM	OT Bathing
9:30 AM	OT Dressing
10:00 AM	OT ADL (KD)
10:30 AM	
11:00 AM	Bowling
11:30 AM	Bowling
12:00 PM	
1:00 PM	PT(AI)
1:30 PM	PT(AI)
2:00 PM	SCI Ed.
2:30 PM	SCI Ed.
3:00 PM	
3:30 PM	OT ADL (KD)
Discharge Date	
OT:	Kim
PT:	Amy
RT	Matt

V

1st time
bowling

Bowling in a wheelchair.

I thought of my dad, got sad, and chuckled at the same time. I was super excited and started to feel that if I was to be in this wheelchair for the rest of my life, I could make it fun, I could be grateful, and I would be active. I knew that my parents were with me in spirit, and that their presence, then and now, was helping me to accept and embrace whatever God had planned for me.

I started to realize I could still live my best life; I just needed to make some changes.

In mid-March, our little group of six from the spinal cord unit went to out on a field trip. I was excited and nervous at the same time. We headed to lunch to a popular restaurant off campus. Several therapists were with us for our safety, but I had to maneuver my wheelchair on and off the van. I paid attention to the others, watching what they did, and didn't do. When it was my turn, I was able to get on and off okay - in the sense that I actually accomplished it, yet, it was a struggle for me considering my neck brace and limited ability to move.

That day I learned being in a wheelchair did not stop my life. I just needed to scope out entry ways and paths to make sure I had enough room for my wheelchair. It got easier every time I went out. Later in the month, Ginger and I went on an outing to the movies and lunch. It was great. We chatted all day long, and maneuvering was much easier. With each outing, my confidence was growing, and I was feeling more and more comfortable in my wheelchair.

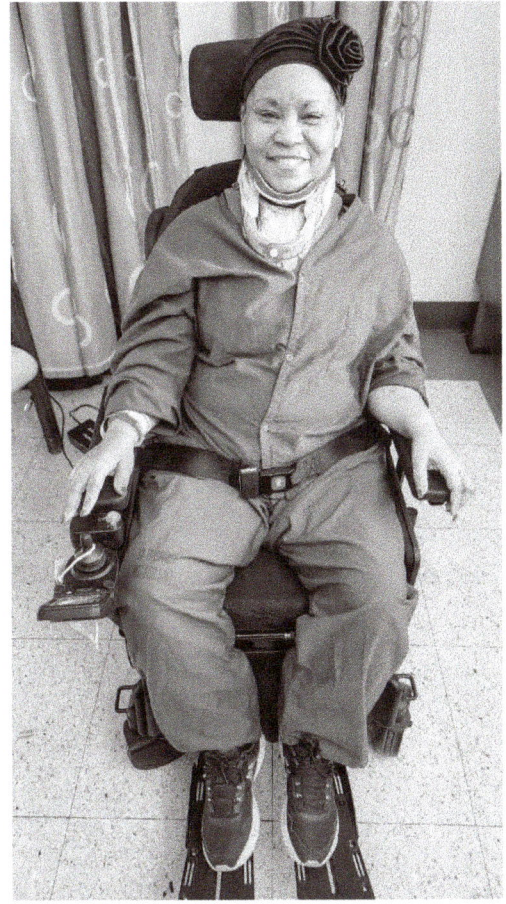

Head covering, neck brace, wheelchair and a smile.

I Was Progressing More Quickly Than Any Of Us Imagined

I learned from Barry that my initial home discharge date was to be in December of 2024, which would be nearly a year from when my spinal cord injury first happened. I was shocked when I heard that because I only remember June 30th as my target date. *Did I hear it but ignore it, and focused on getting out of rehab? I honestly don't know.* Nonetheless, I was tackling every task and situation

53

put before me with the support of my whole team (my hospital team, family and God).

The first home visit is typically scheduled about 90 days before discharge so that the OT/PT team can do an assessment of the environment, make recommendations, and so that the family or facility can prepare for the person's needs. My first home visit was on March 14, 2024.

When we arrived, I was excited when I saw our little townhouse, thrilled to be home with My Love!

They lifted me into the house in my wheelchair because there's a step at the front door. I roll into the living room and chat with My Love while the team counts the steps, and measures the hallways, and each room. They noted that the bedrooms are upstairs, the full showers are upstairs as well, and that we have tall kitchen cabinets. They didn't say too much to Barry or I during the visit, they just allowed us to enjoy each other's company. We spent two hours at my home, I had a small bite lunch instead of minced and moist; and I was back in PT for my 1 pm session.

At 2 pm, I headed downstairs for a Spinal Cord Injury (SCI) Education class. All the while I'm wondering how I am going to function/get around in our townhouse. I spent the rest of the afternoon and evening trying not to worry, and quite frankly, praying for some miracle to happen, knowing we would all be meeting the next morning to speak about accommodations.

PT/OT states the obvious; my home needs a stair lift to get me up and down the stairs. The bathrooms are small and my wheelchair is too wide for that space. I will not be able to reach the kitchen cabinets, and NOTHING in my home will work. It was hard to hear, and it was true.

So the question to my husband is, *"Are you willing to move?"*

"Am I willing to move out of our home and into a new one in like in the next 60 days? A move takes months to plan. And something this specific would take time and research. No. I'm not willing to move."

My younger sister chimes in and states, "Then my sister is coming to Alabama with me until you figure it out."

Oh my, what just happened? Silent tension filled the line.

Finally someone states, "Let's see how we can work this out."

My Love is such a planner. The thought of him having to rush and do it? That would just be too much. I also kinda knew my sister would clap back. She wanted me to be comfortable and safe, and she would move heaven and earth if she could. Actually both of them would, but not our home in 60 days! Though both of them were in the military, My Love is so analytical and has to process everything.

I didn't know the solution in those tense moments, yet, my mind was all over the place. I take the rest of the day to process. My husband and sister only want what's best for me. I knew I would speak with Teres offline and help her to understand that I had to stay close to my doctors and with my husband. I began to pray.

By the time I finished therapy for the day, and after dinner, I decided to let go of my concerns and focus on the one area I could actually control. I decided once again to trust God and my husband. I knew that somehow, someway, this would work out, and there would be peace as well as a way for me to function in my own home.

The next day, March 15th, OT/PT calls another meeting. My Love, my sister and my daughter are on the call. We listen to the plan

OT/PT has created. They want to order a smaller wheelchair, and request permission from the property manager to have a stair lift installed in our townhouse. They want me to have a smooth transition home and believe that we can configure our townhouse to accommodate my needs. During the call, cool heads prevail and we all agree, I'm going home in a smaller wheelchair.

***

After My Home Visit My Body Starts To Spark

In PT, you're working your whole body, mainly the lower body. After a spinal cord injury and being in bed for weeks on end, you have to work through the numbness, tingling and spasms to see if your body wakes up. However, when you're doing that, you cannot feel your extremities - but you're doing it anyway. It's like your brain is telling your extremities to move - your brain and body are not talking and the spinal cord has to heal enough for them to start talking again. The spinal cord is the conductor between your brain and the rest of your body.

Before any therapy I had to stretch, which takes 15-20 minutes. Especially in the beginning, when I was completely unable to move my body, Kat, my therapist stretched me. Stretching was/is essential, especially for a body that doesn't naturally move. Daily I was riding the bike, from my wheelchair. My feet were placed in the bike pedal stirrups and velcroed in. The machine moves the feet. So though my brain was not registering to my body that my legs were in motion (since I could not feel anything), my muscles were being used and exercised. This is how I experienced each activity until I actually regained feeling.

I would also do leg presses, leg curls and use the calf machine. To help me stand I was put in a harness so PT could hold onto me and sit me down if needed. By this time, my arms were working, I could feel them, and I had built up enough strength to wheel my wheelchair in between two parallel bars. I placed my hands on the bars and tried to lift myself to a standing position. In the beginning, the machine was bearing all the weight.

The first few times, I could not stand as my legs were still *Jello*. Then a few more days would go by, and I would try again. In time, I was able to squeeze my butt muscles and stand for a few seconds. It took a few times before I could actually stand on my own. After that, it was on... go baby go! My body knew what I needed to do in order to stand and march in place.

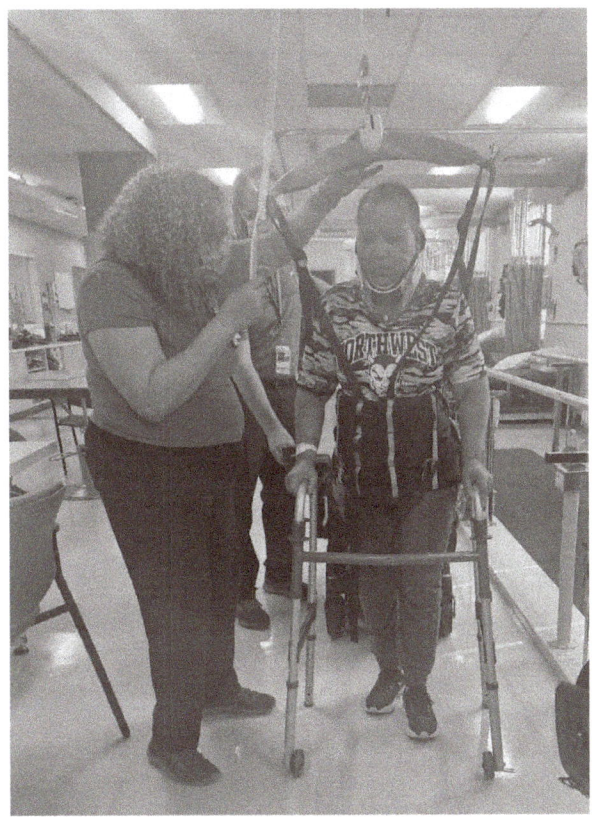

My body is sparking!

A Few Days Later

On some days I would practice writing in OT. When I started, my handwriting was very difficult to read, but it got better with practice. Eventually they added Art Therapy to my afternoon schedule where I would paint and use clay. Led by Laura, the classes were so enjoyable, with snacks and music in the background, everyone was chatting, working and having a good time. Painting brought back old memories for me. I loved drawing and being in class gave me time to reconnect with my artistic side. Don't get me wrong, I'm not very good at drawing but I could look at the examples and follow instructions to finish a project to my own satisfaction. Again, I thought it was fun, but it took a minute to realize it was using my fine motor skills to complete each project... very clever therapy.

One night after another long day, I had a dream. In it, I saw myself walking out of JB. It was strange. I was a bit alarmed. *Is this going to happen months or years from now?* I was not sure of the timing of this walk, yet, I decided to trust. I told God, "I am planning to bling out my wheelchair with crystals and hot pink wheels! However, if Your desire is for me to walk out of here instead of roll, I'll take it! Thank you God!"

Motivated and reinvigorated by that dream, I'm working my butt off in therapy. My legs have been like *Jello* when I try to stand, but I keep pushing, listening and praying.

Then something clicked, I could feel my legs and feet. A few days after they were in the midst of planning our home reconfiguration, I stood in therapy!

I stood, praise God! Then the next day, I stood and could march in place! I was still in the harness and wearing my neck brace. It was hard to see my feet over the brace, but I was doing it!!!

I can tell by the looks on everyone's faces - they have been hopeful for my recovery - yet, in that precious moment, we all knew, we were witnessing a miracle!

Everyone in therapy is cheering! I'm crying! Amy, my PT tech is almost in tears! It's a GOOD day! My progress was added to my chart, and by the time I made it downstairs from therapy, there is chatter everywhere.

"Did you hear Ms. Cooksey took some steps today?" "Yes! She's stepping and marching!"

In my case, once my brain and body were communicating, muscle memory took over. After that day, each afternoon in PT, I would walk the parallel bars; then one day I slowly turned around and walked the other way. I asked to walk without the harness and they were hesitant to let me do it, but gave in. I was so glad to be out of that thing! I continued stepping.

On March 22nd I have more feeling in my feet. *I began walking with a walker!!!*

"What?

"Like how?"

"What did you say?"

"She's walking!"

One of the nurses even brought me artificial flowers to attach to decorate my walker! That was so sweet and motivating.

Without getting too excited, I know walking with a walker is GREAT! But, I have steps at home. *Lord have mercy, can I do this? Can I do this?*

More therapy… another week in therapy… Amy, my PT, calmly states, "Let's see if you can climb a step." *Lord help me! This girl is going to kill me!*

I said, "Okay Amy." I was shaking in my tennis shoes, but I was willing. Trust and believe all precautions were taken, I was hooked up to a lift machine in the ceiling, which is on a track. Even if I slipped, the harness would catch me. I stepped, as if I was stepping into pants. I did not fall! As a matter of fact, I climbed three steps!

Amy was so cute, smart and challenging. She was impressed, but reminded me once again, "The first time is a fluke. Let's see if you can do it again." I did it. Three more steps.

"Let's do it a third time so everyone can see." Lol! Yes a crowd had formed - and her tactics worked every time. By the end of therapy, after climbing three steps three times, I was exhausted, yet felt proud, shocked and excited! It was amazing, just watching God work through me. Just amazing.

Yes, it was 'only' three steps, but I was sweating like I had run a full marathon. I went from being completely paralyzed to stepping up steps, three times three! *Perhaps somehow, some way, my dream will foretell my near future!* I slept like a baby that night, grateful and hopeful.

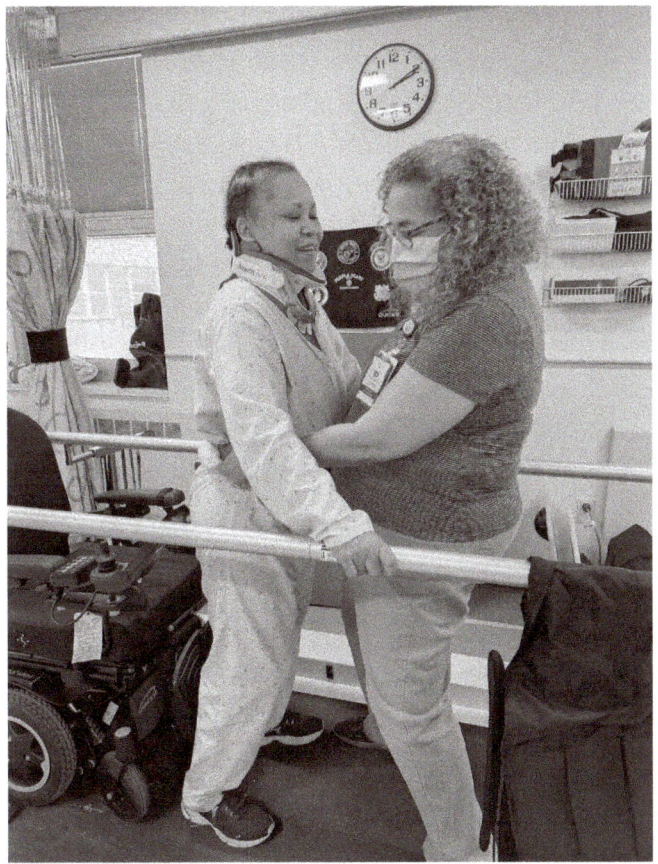

Getting more comfortable.

Mastering The Basics

Everything I had ever done, I had to relearn. Things we take for granted like feeding ourselves, signing our signature, washing ourselves, even shaving, grooming our hair, and putting on compression socks take so much effort and practice to learn again. Although I was standing, I couldn't stand long enough to take a shower... as I got stronger and feeling started coming back, I was able to use shower tools like the grab bar and removable shower head to assist me with washing my back and shaving my legs.

Learning to use the commode again was exciting! For all those months, I had been using a catheter and was on a bowel program (they had to physically "make my bowels work" daily). As my body was reawakening, my bodily sensations were as well. Eventually, I could tell when I had to go. And then I was able to wait and not go; controlled urination and bowel movements were huge victories.

Enjoying The Sun

When I had visitors on the weekends they would give me inspiration and encouragement to keep going. Sometimes, weather permitting, we would sit outside and talk, as getting Vitamin D was good for the soul. Oh the joy of being outside, yes, sunshine, birds, squirrels and good conversation! One of those days, outside in the full sun, I realized I was sluggish after about 20 minutes. I went into the shade, felt better, and headed out to the sun again. Then I was exhausted and needed to rest so I headed to my room to grab some water, tilt and take a quick nap.

The nurse came in to check my vitals and my temperature was around 103. We discussed how I was feeling and my body's response when being in the full sun versus the shade. We realized my temperature gauge was off, as my body was not regulating heat properly. As much as I like to lay out in the sun at the beach or by the pool, they told me I would need to wear a hat and stay out of the direct sunlight going forward.

Real Food, Again

Around this same time as the sun revelation, I graduated to Level 7 on the Minced and Moist Menu. I was so ready for my first real meal! However, before I knew it, one of the nurses had politely cut up everything to bite sized bits!!! I had not asked her to cut up my food! *Geez! May I please eat my chicken tenders and French fries like regular people?*

Let me tell you this was a SLOW process. Each level had to be cleared by my swallow team. Getting from Level 1 to Level 7 was about 8 weeks for me.

Walking That Walk

A gait belt became part of my daily wardrobe after my first attempt to stand. It provided a secure grip for my therapists to guide and support me, just in case I were to fall.

Once cleared by the doctors, I was able to walk the halls of the building, going from my room door to the end of the hallway, maybe 50 feet. It was all measured and recorded each time. I chose to walk on the weekends to keep up my strength. Every other weekend, the PT gym was open. We could go up and exercise. Then Matt, who was the activity director among other things, would open Art Therapy as well. We could work on any projects that were not quite finished.

A few weeks later, the team decided I could try walking outside. I was super excited for this new adventure. Before going out, my PT assistant Lars and I talked about the different terrains I would experience. My first time outside with the walker, I had to practice navigating over cracks in the sidewalk. It had rained the day before, so we practiced in the mud just a little bit to see how to navigate the muddy grass. With each step, we took precautions to ensure I was safe and ready for the challenge. We walked on the sidewalk, and up a small ramp. I got tired. I sat on a nearby bench after each exercise. It takes a lot of energy to walk up a small slope when you've been in a wheelchair for months.

I continued to walk outside. Each day, my distance increased. I became stronger. After I became proficient with my walker, I started picking it up to navigate bumps in the sidewalk. You're not supposed to pick up your walker. Since the walker was getting in my way, the team decided I should graduate to a four-pronged cane. I tried it for a few days. I'm not sure why, but I could not get used to the cane. I asked if I could try walking without any devices.

Amy said, "Sure!"

I did it, and kept doing it! Walking outside was therapeutic for my soul as well. It gave me the confidence to know that if I could walk outside unassisted, I could navigate my home safely. I knew I needed to overcome the staircases if that was to happen. I was focused, and so was Amy.

It's Mid-April...

I was told that I'd needed to go back over to JC, where my journey had begun, to get a second MRI. They needed to check my spine and the placement of my titanium plate in my neck to make sure the screws were still in place.

That morning Laura, my JB nurse called JC and told the radiographer my ride was late and could he please make sure I was seen today.

The tech stated, "Sure! Yes, I remember Ms. Cooksey, I'll do that!"

I heard my nurse say, "The Ms. Cooksey you saw in January is much different than the Ms. Cooksey you will see today. FYI she's walking!!!!!"

I kind of chuckled at their joy in my progress. Sitting on the couch, I continued reading in the waiting area until the EMT came in with a stretcher from the ambulance. Laura rounded the corner and asks the EMT who she's looking for. A bit confused, she says my name.

Laura points to me. The EMT said, "Wow! There's no wheelchair or walker?"

Laura said, "Nope, she's walking without assistance!"

The EMT stated how rare it was for her to transport someone with a spinal cord injury who was walking. We all understood.

I smiled, stood up and thought about how grateful I was to be a walking miracle. Laura and I headed toward the ambulance for our trip. She would assist me with getting in and out of the vehicle, changing into the gown and any other thing I might need. I sat in the front seat to take it all in, the noise, trees everything. I'd been outside in my wheelchair, but this was the first time I'd been able to ride in the front seat and enjoy the view.

We arrived safely to John Cochran and headed to radiology. I checked in, took a seat and waited about 5 minutes for my name to be called. The radiographer smiled so BIG when he saw me. He remembered me, and I remembered him. He was amazed at my progress. I changed into the gown and headed out to the machine. We chatted for 15 minutes while I filled him in on all that had happened since my last visit. The last time he saw me in January, I was completely paralyzed. He and the other nurses had to lift me from my hospital bed to the MRI table.

After the MRI, I changed back into my civilian clothes and chatted with the tech again before leaving. I left JC praying that he saw God's work in me. I was also hopeful that the results would be positive, and that I could finally remove my neck brace permanently. It was a good day.

After reading the results of my MRI, the doctors told me I could remove my neck brace. They told me that my neck would likely be sore in the beginning, while my body was adjusting to not wearing it. They also gave me instructions about neck movement to protect myself. I was very excited and nervous at the same time - I felt free but hesitant, afraid I would injure myself again. *Inside, I also felt if I injured myself again, I didn't know if I could make it.*

Aqua Therapy

Once I had gained my strength and endurance they allowed me to participate in Aqua therapy a few times, which I really enjoyed. It uses all of your body's muscles and is great exercise. One hour of intense aqua therapy fees like five hours of PT/OT. I was able to walk into the pool on my own, very carefully and down the steps.

Though Ginger was discharged before I was, we aqua therapy together, along with my buddy Scott. Led by our instructor Matt, there were blocks we had to step over, then sideways, then step up, step down and then do a squat. After we did that, we put on life vests, and Matt would take us to the deeper side of the pool for leg work - scissors, floating and kicking our feet.

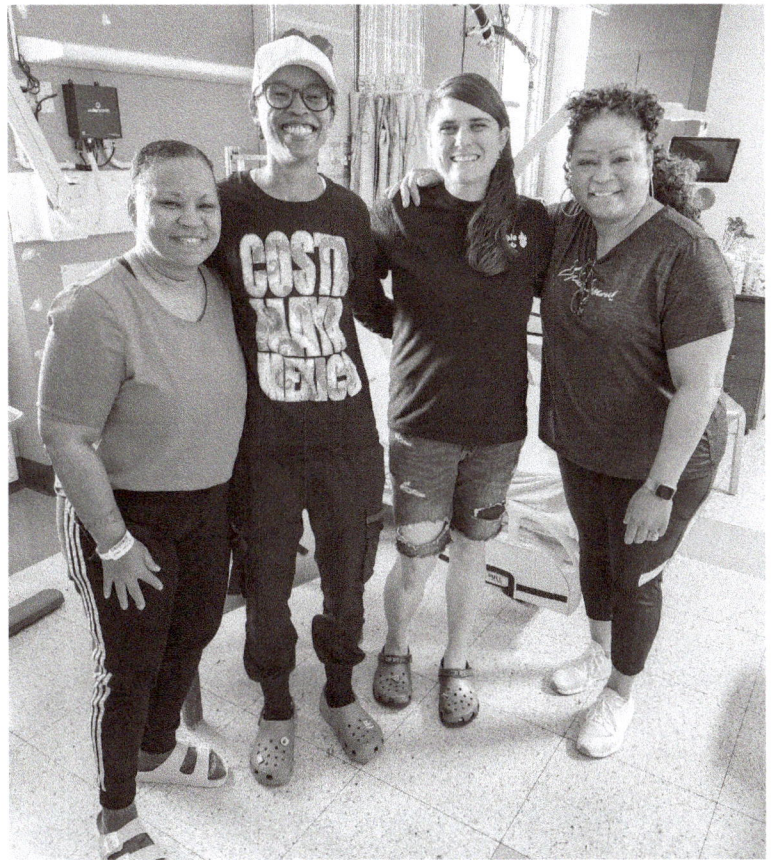

Lisa, Amber, Haylee and Teres. Almost home!

Ringing The Bell

The day I was discharged, there was a bell ringing ceremony. All of my team lined up on both sides of the hallway. They shouted, clapped, cheered and cried as I danced my way down the line and rang the bell.

Ringing the bell had me on an emotional rollercoaster. I was happy, sad and anxious all at the same time. I was definitely happy to be going home. I missed My Love; I wanted to be with my husband.

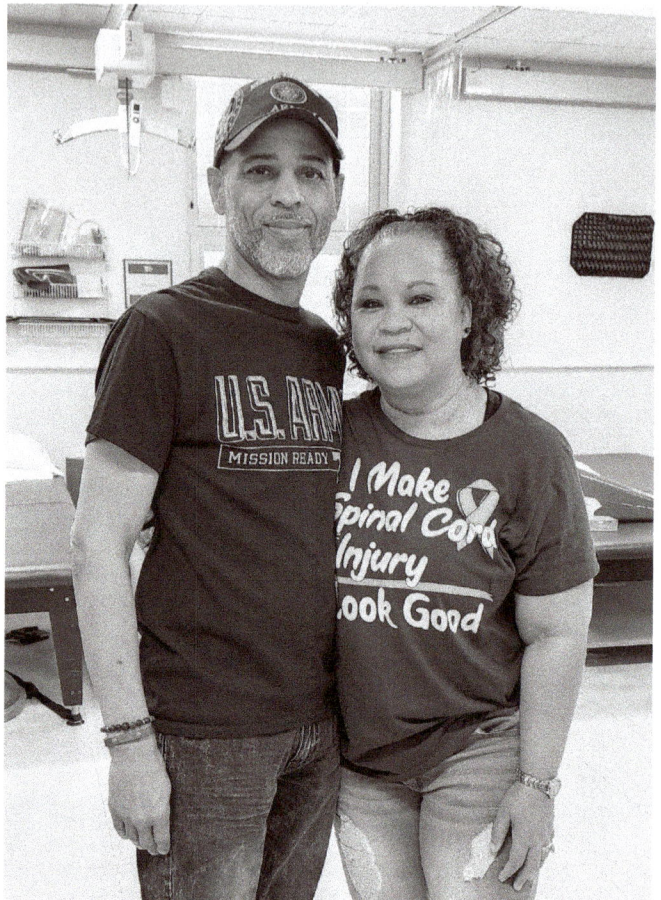

Barry and I shortly before I was discharged.

I was sad because I knew being outside with the rest of the world and not in my protected bubble could be dangerous. Fear of being bumped, losing my balance, falling and not being able to get up scared me.

And, I was anxious to see what I could do. I was thinking about all of the chores I needed to do. Would I be able to stand at the stove and cook? Could I still be productive and be an asset to my household? Would I be able to go back to work?

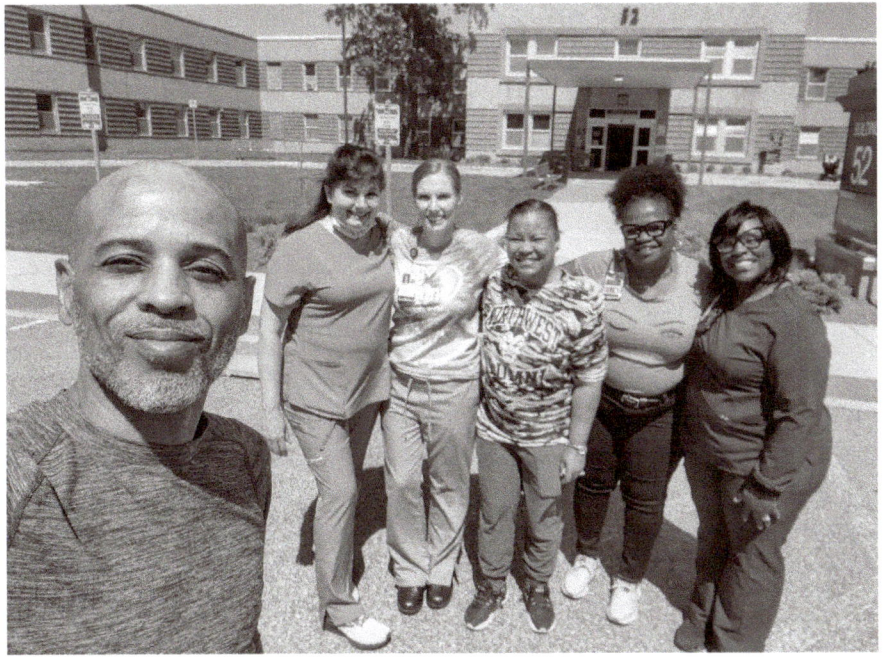

Protected, with part of the team.

There were so many unknowns, yet, I was looking forward. I was looking forward to getting back to my life, to hanging out, to painting, to line-dancing and to loving my life -outside.

Being Home Is...

*Fantastic and challenging
at the same time.*

The first week I only had the energy to only sleep and eat. I'm sure you'll understand this statement....you are NOT able to rest while in the hospital. So being home, I needed to rest and sleep.

Now after that first week, I was ready to take on the world. I quickly realized I needed extra time to do everything i.e. my daily chores such as vacuuming, washing dishes, cleaning the kitchen, cooking etc. I needed to rest and take breaks often. My journey took a turn when I realized I was not living in my protected bubble any longer. At JB, someone was always there to lend a hand or show me an alternate way to complete a task. At home, it was all me trying to figure things out except when I allowed My Love to help me. Yes, I have remained independent, though I am getting better with asking. In some aspects, I wanted to try whatever first then ask for help if needed. I wanted the old Lisa back, this 2.0 version of myself was driving me crazy.

I'm not complaining, God brought me through the fight of my life, and I'm sure by now you know exactly how I feel about God. It's just this new me is different. It's taking time to get used to her. Walking up and down the two flights of stairs five or six times in a couple hours is draining. Now I've become strategic in how I move and plan my day accordingly.

When I get up, I do a 5-minute bible study when I wake up. After I get dressed, I head downstairs to have coffee and breakfast with My Love. Sometimes our conversation is 30 minutes, and sometimes we are sitting and laughing for 3 hours.

Every other day, I head outside for a walk. I turn on my music, stretch first, and then go about a mile, stopping to rest a few times. Once I'm back inside, I normally stretch again while catching the news on TV, and I rest for a little while. After that I'll usually wash any dirty dishes and head upstairs to get cleaned up. Then for an hour or two, I catch up on reading about world news, people and events. If something piques my interest, I do deep dives to learn more, while lounging. Barry might join me for another chat and/or I journal for a while.

A couple of times a week, I meet with my girlfriends to have breakfast, walk the park, catch a movie or go to a concert. I get my 'manis and pedis' every other week, as self-care is very important to me.

Throughout our marriage, Barry and I have celebrated our wedding anniversary monthly. About four months after I got back home, we started celebrating outside again. We enjoy going to the movies, an art museum, having a family game night or checking out live music at the City Winery.

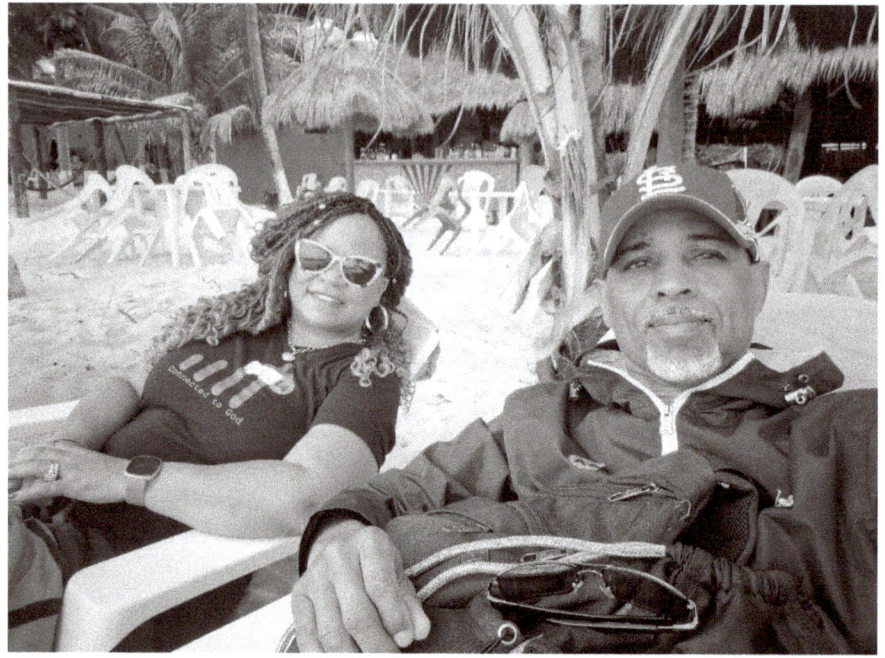

Barry, and I, enjoying the sun.

Of course I could tell you more about my chores like laundry and such, but I won't.

I Continue Stretching And Celebrating

I'm still going to outpatient therapy which helps tremendously, I need the accountability and the structure and I enjoy chatting with Meredith, my PT therapist. She's such a sweet person, yet she pushes me to do my best.

My left side is still weak, in pain and numb, yet I find the strength to go on, and push through in a healthy way to ensure I can still walk and take care of myself without any assisted devices. For a quadriplegic this is HUGE because a severe spinal cord injury and being able to walk unassisted is such an accomplishment.

My back has been tight for some time, and I stretch every morning before getting out of bed. Outpatient therapy staff are constantly showing me different exercises to help with my back issues. Keeping up with my therapy is imperative to my recovery. It's been over a year since my injury. At this point, all of the remaining issues will probably be with me for the rest of my life. I'm thankful to be alive, so having to live with this new me is a privilege. I promise to live my best life from this day forward.

This past winter, my first after my injury, was rough for me. The cold weather made me achy and stiff. I take vitamins and supplements along with a few medications for pain, insomnia and mood, and they did help. Unfortunately, my insomnia medication had a side effect of weight gain. I'm exactly 5 feet tall, and I gained over 40 pounds. The weight gain has taken a toll on my body. I tire easily and feel sluggish. The good news is that we were able to change the medication and I'm already losing a bit of weight. I'm excited about spring and summer, as I can walk more and enjoy the warmth.

I Visited My JC ICU Family

One day before therapy, I visited the ICU to say hello as this team had saved my life on two occasions. Each doctor, nurse and tech that provided care had spoken such positive words to me on a daily basis. They confirmed what God was speaking to my spirit; small daily victories. I saw several of the doctors and members of the staff. Between them and me, there weren't any dry eyes in the hallways. I think seeing me walk gave them the strength to push forward and to know their work and care is an important part of each patient's journey.

Being Lisa 2.0

Today, because of my brain fog, concentration and memory are not as strong as they used to be. And, to be transparent, I may look okay but I'm not. What I mean by that is it takes me forever to shower and get dressed. I can only sit for 15 to 20 minutes at a time until my back begins to throb even more deeply than the pain I experience 24 hours a day. The residual effects of my left-side weakness include tingling and numbing.

I tried to go back to work on June 3, 2024. I had the limitations of only working four hours a day, and was able to take breaks when needed. What I did not anticipate was not being able to do my job. I had such high hopes in the beginning, and quickly realized my accountant skills were pretty much non-existent. I could not figure out how to compute or how I could research any of my daily tasks. Considering accounting is such a fast-paced environment, within six weeks, I realized I had to resign.

My neurology team told me I would be a good candidate to start the disability process, which was a challenge for me because that wasn't the plan I had for myself.

You see, I had "retired" right before Covid 19, as it was always my goal to retire at 57 years old. It had worked out well, as my position moved to Maryland and I was not willing to move there, so I decided to retire, and I was "good" with retirement.

My Love had been retired from the military and then post office for about five years, so I was excited to join him on the journey. I made time to study my Bible and to start walking almost daily, eating better, and lost over 25 pounds in the process. We loved going to Creve Coeur Park together where he could ride his bike while I walked. Sometimes we ventured to Forest Park as well.

I laugh as I remember us going to Walmart, and me picking out a little pink Huffy bike for $95, planning to join him with his $500+ "bike extravaganza." It had been 40 years since I'd ridden. Instead of starting off at the park, we started riding around in circles in our neighborhood for practice. My Love has always been my encourager. Every other day we would ride a little further until I could build up my confidence. Eventually we went on longer rides in both parks. Sometimes I would walk, and other times I would ride my bike. It just depended on the day and how I felt. During most of Covid, we had family game night with just the two of us. There was a lot of *Battleship*, backgammon, checkers and a little *Monopoly*. Being retired was great.

Toward the end of Covid, My Love and I took a five day Caribbean cruise with my sister and brother-in-law, and that was great. I enjoyed all of the quality time the pandemic and retirement afforded. We had laughed, enjoyed movies and snuggling on the couch.

It all felt great, yet, I thought I had more to give, so I decided to go back to work. In my previous position I had been a senior accountant/manager with lots of responsibility and 12 direct reports. When I decided to rejoin the workforce, I found an individual contributor position where I could work with people, but not have to endure the stresses that come with leadership and the challenges of being a woman in the accounting field.

I felt there were more young women I could mentor. I have always believed my life's purpose to be teaching - and mentoring allows me to give back. I don't think there are enough Black women accountants - and I wanted them to see me and know it is possible.

I had planned to work a few more years, and retire. God decided otherwise.

My memory issues will be with me for the rest of my life. Getting used to my new normal is probably the hardest part of this journey. I'm still trying to love and accept Lisa 2.0. I'm still standing only by God's grace and mercy. I don't have enough words to express how I feel about the nurses, doctors and techs who helped me along the way, I'm forever grateful to them and my family.

Amber Shares

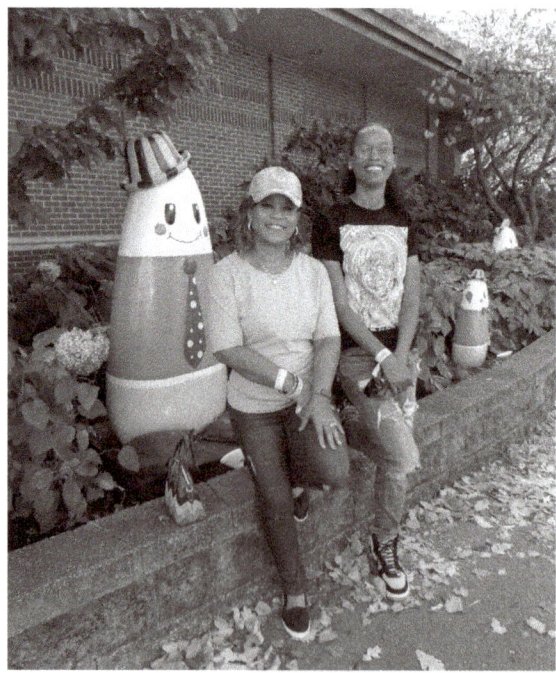

Mom and daughter.

Amber, My Daughter Had Been A Medic In The United States Army. I think she was confused and angry because my injury caught her off guard, just like the rest of us. I'm thankful for her support, and that she was able to drop everything and come check on me. She was so nurturing, loving and caring. Also, being present, asking questions I didn't know I needed answers to, was so helpful.

A year ago today, I got the call my mom was in the hospital. I filled a backpack with a change of clothes and my iPad, and flew 1,700 miles to find out what the f*ck was going on.

When I arrived in Missouri, I realized how much colder the Midwest winter hits than the California sunshine. I was ill prepared not just mentally, but apparently physically too. My stepdad picked me up from the airport, and we went straight to the hospital.

The ICU was a strange place to be. Seeing my mom in a hospital bed with tubes up her nose was a strange place to be. Life was really strange and hard to understand. (Have you ever seen your hero hit by kryptonite?)

We found out she had to have one surgery... and then another. Her first surgery went well. They were hopeful she would regain the ability to move her arms and legs, but walking...

Well, "We can't know what your recovery will look like."

And then it got worse. She was alert. Stay alert, stay alive. She was talking with us. Then, mid conversation, she stops.

The nurses rush in "Lisa, Lisa can you hear me?" She didn't.

They rushed my stepdad and I out of the room and... I thought that would be the last time I ever saw her. The last time I got to hear her voice, the last time I held her hand.

We prayed in the waiting room. But thank God, Allah, the stars and the spaghetti monster because she made it back to us.

And because she's a hero, she relearned how to move and walk. She's not the same as she was, but she's still here.

But the lesson I want to share comes after this story. Despite almost losing my mom, then losing my grandfather and grandmother four months apart, I have been living life like it's promised.

I take that sh*t for granted, that tomorrow is going to resemble today, or last week.

I think we have to be wired this way to maintain our narrative, our sense of order. Because if we really counted all the ways we could be offed each day well... we would all probably become agoraphobes, also, afraid of our homes.

I haven't figured out the solution to this one yet. I know that mindfulness, journaling, and presence help. Yet, holding onto the idea that tomorrow isn't promised but living like it is, that's tough.

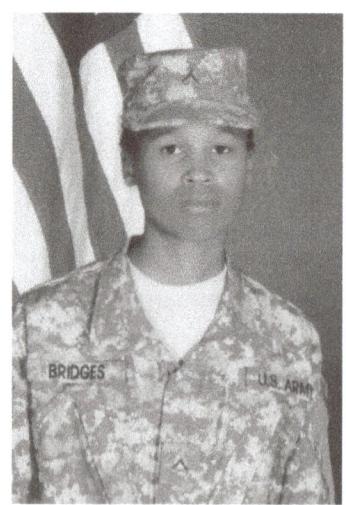

Loving daughter, Amber.

Mental Health Struggles Affect the Majority Of Us

If you don't acknowledge pain and trauma in your life, you won't heal. You'll have a hard time finding your purpose and being Victorious!

From The Beginning We Began Addressing My Mental Health

A psychiatrist was part of my team. Before my spinal cord injury, when I was seeing a counselor for my PTSD, I was very hesitant. I knew I had to open up and be vulnerable - so she could hear and see the areas I needed help. In our very first meeting we were talking and she said, "I believe you." That was all it took - just someone to believe me. Because sometimes people don't believe you or don't want to believe you. But her having experience talking to other veterans, she knew my story was true, and that provided comfort to me.

The Mental Struggles

I struggled quite a bit with nightmares, insomnia, hallucinations and chronic pain. Only by God's grace and therapy and a few medications have I been able to see my way back to a healthy and stable mental state. I smiled and thanked God daily. It's really hard to talk about. I don't' want you to pity me or feel sorry for me. Trust me when I say I'm so much better. It's part of the journey. A very hard part of my journey. I would wake up from a nightmare scared, heart pounding, screaming or crying. Yet not remembering what the nightmare entailed at times just paralyzed me with fear. Being paralyzed left me helpless in a sense; I'm there in that bed not able to defend myself.

My ego doesn't want to let me go that personal.

The spinal cord injury is one thing, but the mental piece is another. It's been a dark journey. It has taken me to a place where I've had to fight my way back - literally laying and praying and crying and fighting my way out of those nightmares - and I know part of it is because of my PTSD from the military. The spinal cord injury on top of it opened some old wounds, put them front and center, and beat down my spirit. I've literally had to tell myself every day, *You survived, there is no one here you have to fight, and God's going to keep you.* It'll never be over. But I am better equipped to cope with it through counseling, and telling myself those positive affirmations every day.

I don't feed myself false narratives. Sometimes our brains tell us something that's not true, like, "I'm never gonna get better." *Nope.* It will open up a whole can of worms, and this story cannot be about that!

What are the true narratives? I am getting better every day. It's a slow process, I'll never be the old me - but the new me is healing and getting comfortable in my own skin again.

Some Ways Counseling Is Helping

The isolation, the fear and feeling like I'm not a whole me... these are the thoughts I fight to overcome daily.

Seeing the bigger picture - dissecting the lies and telling myself the truth.

Move better in crowds - I can be very oversensitive, and I know now I have to arrive early, check out my surroundings, make sure I'm comfortable - because it can heighten my anxiety when I'm around a lot of people.

It's okay not to be okay - to talk it out with a counselor, to work through it, to know that every day is not going to be peaches and cream, and some days you'll have to take a break, check in with yourself, and if you just need a little time to yourself to regroup, then it's okay to take the time to regroup.

Trusting people again. I think we tend to put 'everybody and all' in our sentences; - everybody is bad and all people suck. Counseling allows you to take away the 'all' and put in 'some' or a 'few'.

And it's a beautiful part of the healing process - to find a counselor who connects with you, takes the time to help you see things in a different light, and one that gets to know you.

Sometimes when I'm typing, I'm so deep down in my feelings, it's hard to flush it out. But I think, talking about it with someone I trust makes it better. I know sometimes I'm really hard on myself.

For Those Who May Resist Counseling: Give it a chance. There is this dysfunctional stereotype we have about counseling, and I think it's unhealthy. I feel like if God made doctors to help heal our bodies, of course he made doctors/therapists to help heal our minds.

Dealing With Post Traumatic Stress Disorder (PTSD)

PTSD has triggers, so learning what triggers you is part of the healing process.

When you look back on those triggers, you will see how it affected every aspect of your life.

And when you discover how it affected every aspect of your life through counseling, don't beat yourself up. You can't go back and change it. Your job from this point on is to continue healing and move forward. If the opportunity arises for you to go back to a person and apologize, definitely take the chance. Go back, and apologize. And if there's no opportunity, be okay with it. Part of it is making peace with yourself.

If you're dealing with a person that has PTSD, know that there will be some good times and some not-so-good times, but it's worth the fight for you and for them.

Trauma Often Happens In The Home, But Goes Unchecked

Seeking help is the best thing you can do to break some of those generational curses.

Mothers: Just because your mom had boyfriends in and out does not mean you have to have boyfriends in and out.

Daughters: When you saw your dad beat on your mom does not mean you allow your boyfriend to beat on you - that is not love.

About Sons: Mom's can baby their sons a bit too much, and don't allow the fathers to be a bigger influence - sometimes wanting to keep their sons for themselves. Sons need the male presence and development for guidance - to allow them to be successful.

Fathers: Go get the counseling that's needed - you are destroying your families when you leave your daughters and sons looking to other male figures to fill the void that you left - you're leaving young sons to be the head of the household when they don't have the capacity, knowledge, skillset, money, resources to carry the burden that is not theirs to carry.

It's sad; it leaves everybody broken and searching for unhealthy ways to cope with life. So many turn to abuse - alcohol, food, drugs, porn... Go get the help that's needed. Don't be afraid. Don't let your ego get in the way of seeking help.

It will take patience, effort, understanding, gentleness, love, faith and the willingness to continue practicing these things every single day to heal and to maintain *Hope and Perserverance on your journey to being Victorious.*

Why I Joined The Military

I was frustrated and tired of college - just restless - and my dad had some really good experiences he'd shared. He always inspired me and told me it was okay to dream bigger than St. Louis - and to go explore it; don't stay here like your friends. So going off to college helped me see bigger than St. Louis, and then when I got restless, I thought the military would be a good place to start a career.

How Can One Suffer From PTSD?

Trauma has nothing to with combat. Trauma can be something that happened to you, happened to someone else ... so many situations can lead you to experience PTSD. You were harassed in such a way that you feared for your life, which could be true or not true, but your brain perceives it as true - and that can be a trigger for PTSD.

You could have seen someone being assaulted physically, and that can also lead to a diagnosis of PTSD. The traumatic piece and the stress piece isn't about combat. There are plenty of people out here in the world that may suffer from PTSD and not even know it.

Seeing your dad beat your mom can lead to PTSD for everyone involved. So don't be afraid to acknowledge what you're feeling, going deeper within yourself and asking for help is the way you get to wholeness - and you want to be a whole you - mentally, spiritually, physically and financially are some ways you become a whole you.

Reflections

A Woman's Point Of View

> *"Being a member of the military can be beneficial and complex."*

My Dad Theodore

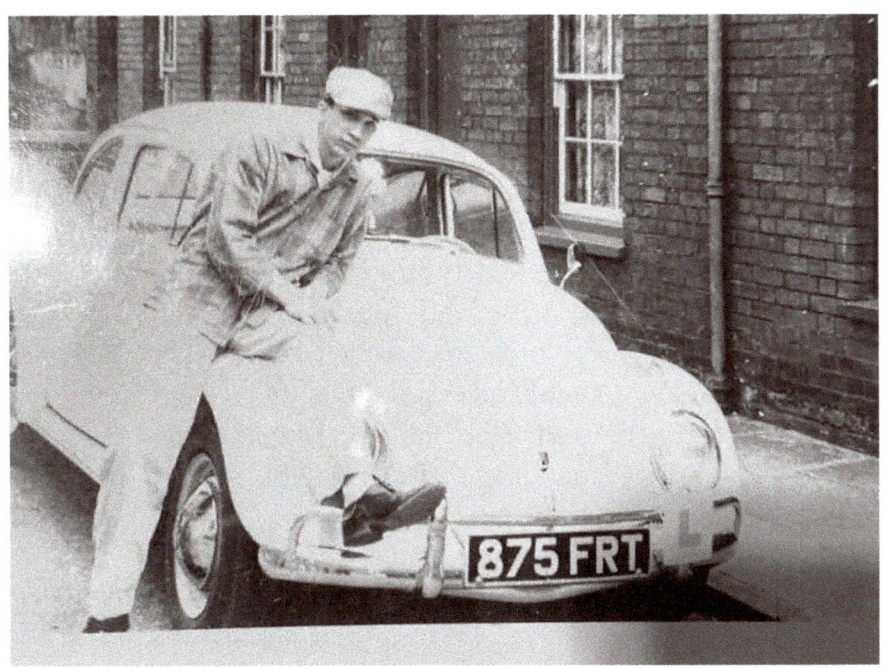

Dad, Theodore.

My Dad painted a great picture of the military...

The travel, the comradery, the ability to earn a living, to have a great career and the respect for the American flag. Yet, what he could not warn me about was the culture of the military and how women were treated. Being on active duty in the mid 80's was a struggle.

I enlisted hoping to make the military a career, a 20 year career. I knew the road would be tough, physically and mentally. Yet, I quickly learned I would have to fight for equal treatment and for my dignity.

One of the reasons I trained before enlisting was to ensure I was up to the task. BUT, I did not expect the degrading comments, name calling, groping and physical abuse I endured. In the 80's, it appeared this behavior was okay; at times it was swept under the rug, or the individual was transferred to another base quickly without any repercussions or charges being filed. I've spoken to so many ladies that were abused mentally, spiritually and physically.

A positive of my Veteran experience was becoming friends with Ginger at a time when my life and hers were hanging in the balance. To this day, we still talk on a weekly basis. We experienced so much together, I simply have no words. Ours is a friendship I will treasure for the rest of my life. We laughed, cried, watched movies, and danced our way through rehab, first in our wheelchairs, and now on our feet!

Though I don't regret enlisting, I'm not sure that much has changed in terms of the culture and treatment of women in the military. If you or another woman you know is choosing that path, I have three pieces of advice.

My Advice To ANY Woman Considering The Military Is To:

1. Protect yourself at all times
2. Never go anywhere alone
3. Surround yourself with other ladies that will have your back

The discipline is a life-long gift which will help you in the military and your civilian life.

The "I can do it attitude" and "I've been trained on what to do" line of thinking will keep you motivated, and successful.

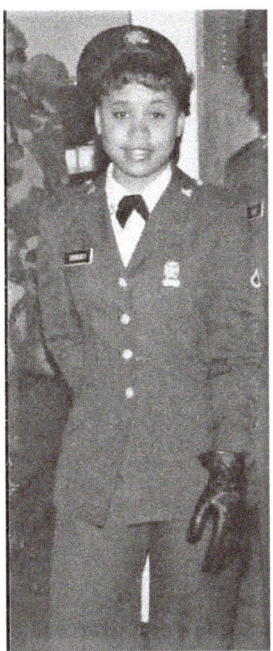

Private First Class Cooksey.

Your experiences will build perseverance, honor and self-respect, and this will help you in any career you choose after the military.

Impact Of My Injury

I'm sad because I know what my husband went through to the end; and my job as a wife is not to bring pain.

My job is to be Barry's helper, confidant, and that mirror reflection of him. I want him to see God in me, and I see him the same way. So to see him in so much pain weighs heavy on me. I told him a long time ago before we got married (when he had cancer), because he asked me if I still wanted to get married, not knowing if he would survive or not. I told him, I am his ride or die. I will see him through the end.

I think all my life I've been taking care of those I love, God comes first, then my family, then myself. That means it's all about them and never about me. Their well-being - I need to make sure they are okay. And there is nothing I won't do for my family.

It's a balance, I'm so very grateful and thankful; I could never thank God enough. Yet, a piece of me will always feel a certain kind of way about this whole journey. I have to constantly work on me, and accept the new me that is me. Lisa 2.0.

In November 2023 - I was at 100% capacity.

In The Ambulance - Was probably at 5% and didn't know I was one head turn away from being permanently and completely paralyzed from the neck down.

After The Second Surgery - I was hopeful and then everything seemed to crash around me as the doctors fought to bring me back, as I was one heart beat from dying.

Back At Home After Rehab - I was at home early in April, instead of December. I was able to navigate the stairs, and they didn't need to put in the stair lift. They cancelled it! I probably slept 18 hours each day for the first five days. I only ate, slept and showered for a week.

That was a big change for me because in the hospital, I was up at 6am, getting meds, food, then up and going for therapy. I had already made plans to go to outpatient therapy so I could continue to work on getting stronger, which I did. I came home early from therapy because they ran out of things for me to do. They couldn't think of any more challenges, so they told me to go home. It was so fast. The way God moved was so fast.

In March, I came home in my wheelchair for a home visit. Therapy was going so well I began walking the entire JB Campus with my favorite walking buddy, Lars. By the time I was home on April 30th, I was able walk the stairs and do chores as I normally would. It took me a little more time, and I had to spread them out a little more, but I was able to do them. In therapy, they made me wash dishes and do my own laundry. They helped me cook, which prepared me to be ready for life back at home.

Mentally - I'm getting better each day. Talking to my therapist helps me put things in perspective. She helps me dig deeper, stay centered, and not be so hard on myself. Part of me still struggles with thinking there was something I could've done differently. It's almost like "I didn't lose everything, but I felt like I was experiencing some kind of Job moment" - She said I didn't lose everything, so it's not a Job moment. But I lost my ability to be me.

It's devastating not to be able to feed yourself, wash your hair or even write your name. But just like Job, God restored it all.

Physically - I realize I'll never be the same. I won't be that old Lisa who ran the ½ marathon or the old Lisa who was out riding my bike with My Love. I'm cautious now because I'm afraid of hurting myself. One of my concerns is going outside for a walk, falling and not being able to get up. That's really a mental concern, because physically, I can go out and walk, though I can't run.

Living in rehab, in the facility, I was in a protected bubble. Living outside of that protective bubble is a bit scary at times. But I know I can go outside and walk, let them know where I'm going, and turn on my location so they'll know where I am. I can walk and even if I fall. I can physically get myself up. I can do those things - but my confidence is not there, and I want it to be.

Before, I was fearless, wanting to go sky diving out of a plane with a person on my back. Today, I am hesitant because I no longer feel fearless. I want that feeling again. That edgy feistiness - I love that about myself.

I've been thinking and realizing, nothing is impossible for God. I feel rich: Rich in life, rich in my spirit; just rich and full. I'm relieved to see my family whole and healthy because it took a toll on them. I remember my sister telling me that she felt like she couldn't breathe.

My husband and daughter are both slender. My daughter is 5'9" and probably weighs 110 pounds. So to hear and see her now, working on gaining some weight because she wants to be healthy, brings me joy. When I was in the hospital, I don't think they were not practicing self-care; they were too concentrated on me and what I needed. The roles were reversed. They were caring for me instead of me caring for them. And there's nothing wrong with that, though I often feel like there is. I'm always the helper and it's hard for me to accept help, but through this journey, I had to.

Barry and I laugh because in December of 2023, we were saying we were out too much, and said we needed to go and sit down! This sitting down wasn't exactly what we were thinking of or talking about.

Barry, Lisa's Husband

I call her, my beloved wife Lisa, My Beautiful.

My Beautiful wife is a phenomenal person and her smile is radiant. Early on, she asked me to document her journey. So, that's one of the reasons I took pictures of her on the ventilator. Although they told me what to expect before I entered the room that day, I wasn't prepared for what I saw.

She was still with us, and continued making progress, whenever I looked at that picture I got emotional and just cried. Each time I would tell the Lord, "Thank you Lord. And Lord, this is too big for me, you've got to take this. Lord, it is not my desire to lose my wife. I love you Lord, and Your will be done. And please save her."

This was my daily prayer with God during the time she was in Intensive Care. The doctors and nurses were being hopeful but I couldn't really see the improvements, and they had to keep pushing back her rehabilitation because of all of the complications. It was a frightening and vulnerable time for us.

Looking Back, During Hospitalization:

I found myself relying on God more. I was weak, He was strong in me.

You take the vows, and when it comes - it's boots on the ground because her condition came out of nowhere, and I wanted to know why. I thought I was prepared on some things, but I was not - this was my wife.

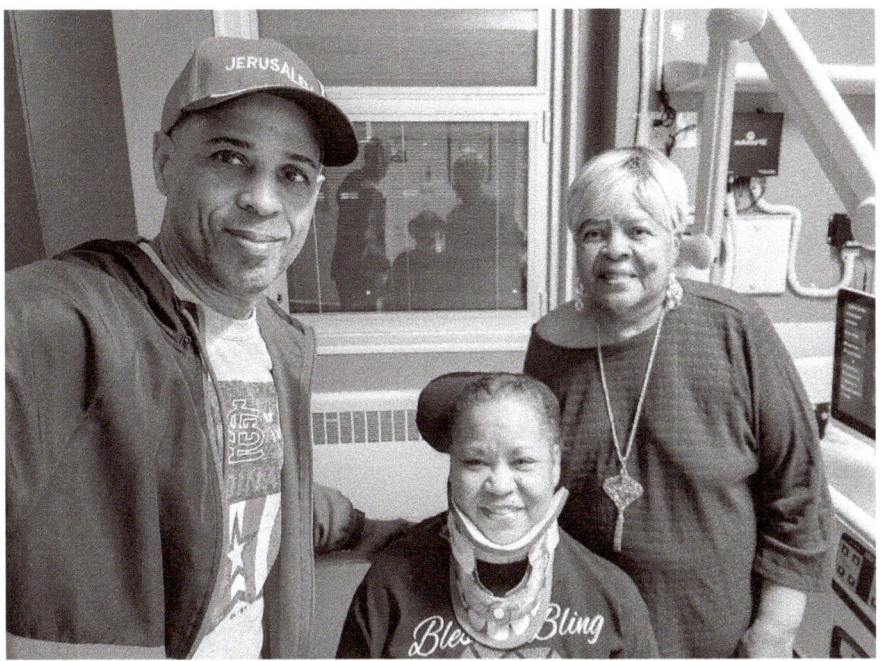

Barry, Lisa and Barry's Mom, Linda.

It was both my wife, and my mother - the love is the same but the relationship are different. My mother's health was failing; my wife's prognosis was decent. Here I was, doing my best to be strong for both of them.

My cousin said, "The enemy came to attack you through your mother and your wife since he could not do it to you directly. Your faith and trust in God are going to get you through this."

I thought, *Me on my own? Without My Beautiful? No!*

Okay Cousin. Yes, I had to rely on God.

I said, "Lord, you didn't bring us this far to call her home." I told myself, *He loves me, He trusts me to be her husband. He got me through 911, Afghanistan, Turkey and prostate cancer and now this? No Lord!*

"Lord, if it is Your will to take her, only You will be able to get me through this. You love me, you protect me. Why not take me?"

Protecting Lisa

Primarily, it was Amber, Teres and I at the hospital when they could be in town. Many people inquired about Lisa's condition; high school alum, members of our church, and many Facebook friends, women and men alike. I was leery. I wanted no drama; no chaos. So, I picked three people to keep informed about Lisa's condition. They spread the word to others, and we were able to streamline who visited; we believed she would walk again, but as you know, getting there was a process.

Day To Day Was Difficult, But I Hid It

Daily supplication with God got me through. When visiting her, I had to sit in the parking lot 30 to 40 minutes before I went into the hospital, crying in the car before I could see her to get myself together. She could see that my eyes were red, but we didn't talk about it; we just enjoyed our time together.

Once or twice she did say, "You don't have to come every day." I responded, "Well, what else am I going to do?"

I missed one day; it was it was April 7th, my birthday. I didn't go out there, and though people were calling, I just literally slept all day. I needed to rest.

Normally, it took 45 minutes or an hour from our house to JB; but the roads were under construction the whole time. There were accidents regularly, and it was very dangerous on HWY 55. The 24 miles took me 1 hour and 45 minutes each way.

When I was driving, I was focused on being safe and reaching My Beautiful.

Some days I would come from the hospital, make it home and not remember how I got there; I was mentally, spiritually and physically exhausted.

When my mother was diagnosed with pancreatic cancer, she did not want to go to a nursing home or come to my home. She wanted to die at home. My mother said, "You can hire someone to take care of me. Go take care of Lisa." They each loved each other so much.

When we weren't sure Lisa could navigate the stairs in our townhouse, of course, I felt like, *This is my wife, and I want to take care of her - Team Beautiful.* I was prepared to put things in storage and set up a bed downstairs. There's a bathroom downstairs. We'd move all of the furniture, and make her comfortable.

Lisa is so loved, Teres felt like, *Hey, that's my sister, I can take care of her.* But, she was out of state. I didn't want to be without my wife; and my mom was in the middle of her illness. I needed her to be home, with me, in our home. We talked about it like my grandmother taught me; with love guiding the conversation, intense fellowship, determined to reach an agreement and understanding, it all worked out.

Thankfully, Lisa came home on April 30th. She was able to go up and down our steps though they had projected it to be December based on her progress at the time.

I believe this happened because of God's grace and mercy, and Lisa's will to do, to live and to get better. God and her got her home sooner. *To God be the Glory!*

I lost my bonus mother on Christmas Day of 2023, and then I lost my biological mother on July 19, 2024. My Beautiful was with me, and we grieved together in the presence of the Lord.

I've shed a couple of tears. Thank you for being patient. It's emotional; this process. It's a lot.

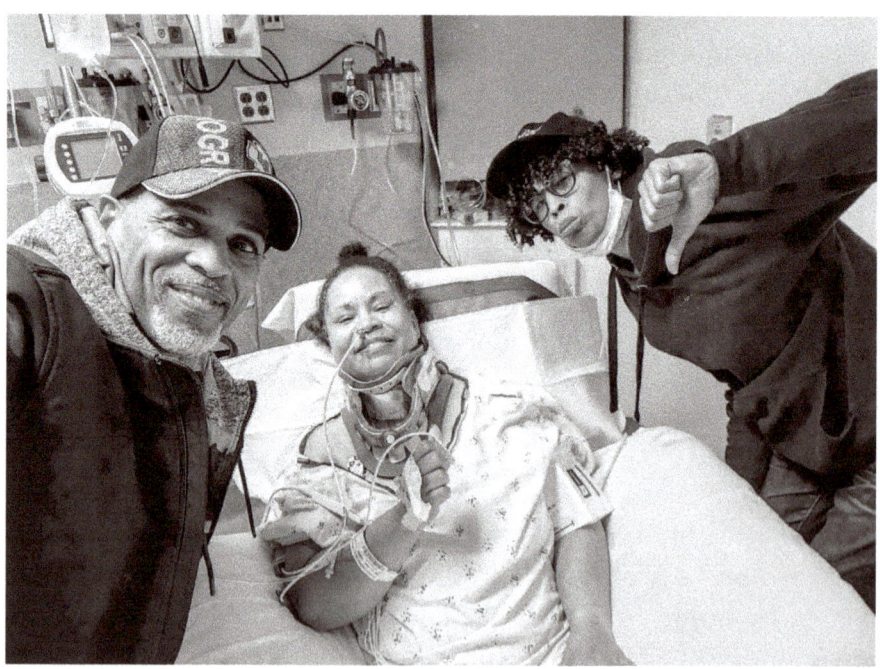

Barry, Lisa and Amber, grateful.

Finding Hope And Perseverance

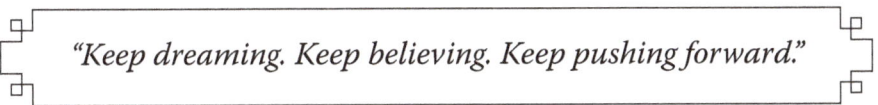

"Keep dreaming. Keep believing. Keep pushing forward."

This journey has taught me that with God's help, I have the strength to make it through any challenge set before me. It took some time to get used to others calling me a walking miracle because I'm not an 'in the spot light' kinda girl. Yet, now I embrace the walking miracle statement and give God the glory each time I speak to someone about my journey.

I know that who I am, what I've accomplished, and the person I continue to strive to be is because of my faith in God. And when you see me, I want you to see God working in my life and in my body because I know that I could not have made it on this journey without Him.

Don't be afraid to challenge the norm when it comes to whatever it is you're setting out to do. Be cautious and understand there are those who are going to downplay you, attack your character, and try to set you up for failure. Let the haters hate. Bring your A Game and make sure you're ready. Don't allow anyone to dampen your dreams. Keep dreaming, keep believing, and keep pushing forward. Be prepared to fight for what God has for you, and you will be *Victorious*.

Resources

Journaling

> *Think it, acknowledge it, write it, reveal it, read it, feel it, forgive it... and then lean into whatever is holding you back in order to move forward to your healing/future.*

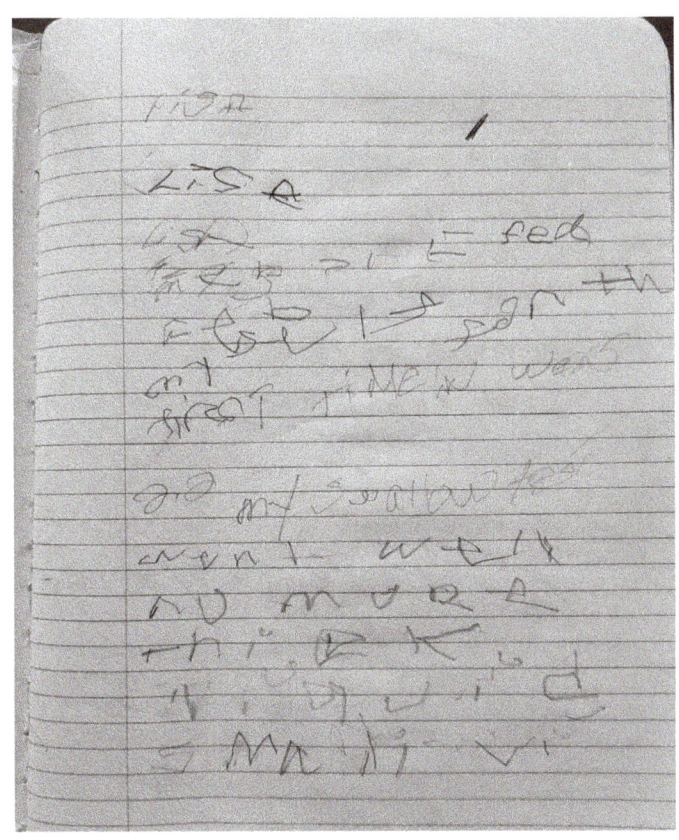

Learning to write again.

Healing Requires Vulnerability

Sometimes we're scared of our own thoughts, but we don't have to be. Putting down on paper (the pain, trauma, or negative experiences from the past) is the start of dealing with what has happened in healthy ways. It's truly a path to healing... When you see it (the past/your thoughts and feelings) in black and white, it becomes real. When we trust ourselves enough to write what we're thinking and feeling, we find the courage and tenacity to see it all the way through.

Forgiveness is one of the biggest, often overlooked things you can do to heal. You have to forgive yourself first, by showing yourself grace. Forgiving somebody else does not mean forgetting or giving them a "free pass." It means you are freeing yourself to move on and heal.

Capturing what's happening in the moment has been a tradition I started when my daughter was a little girl, writing notebooks full of bits and pieces I wanted to share with her. To my surprise, a few days into my rehab, Matt, my therapist, brought me a journal and a pencil with a huge plastic gripper to use. I was excited and sad at the same time; excited because it would help me to write, but sad because at that time, I could not write. The thought of re-learning to write was terrifying. Yet, I was willing to try because I deeply desired to be restored, refreshed, and to have a new start. I want that for you as well.

As you can tell, journaling helped me express myself even when it was not legible. I kept writing, finding peace with each letter. By the time I could actually read what was written, I was enjoying the rhythm of finding small victories daily.

I recommend journaling for everyone and invite you to express yourself, too.

Ms. Lisa's 7 Life Principles To Provide Peace

> *My journey of hope and inspiration is bigger than me.*
>
> For yourself, replace my spinal cord injury with whatever illness or concern you're going through or have experienced in the past; be it mental, physical or spiritual.

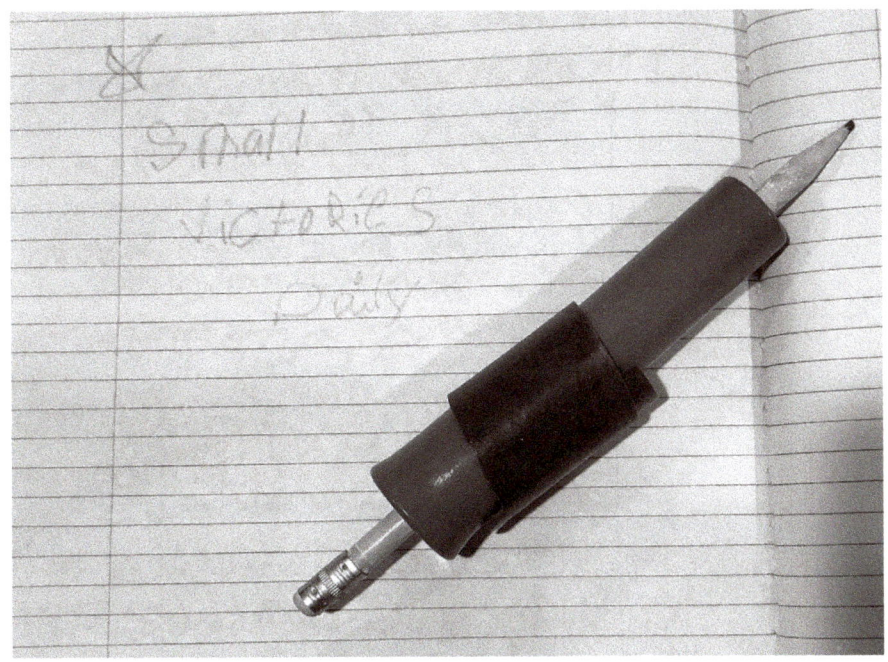

Remember, small victories daily will get you through it all.

During The Darkest Times, Don't Give Up

While recovering in ICU, I was taking a medication that made me hallucinate. It was alarming and very terrifying. I would wake up and see birds on my nose, mice on my blankets and so forth. The first few times this happened, I cried silently and stayed awake. The fourth time, I started to pray. I recited **The Lord's Prayer**, *Matthew 6:9-13*, several times, and fell back to sleep without issue.

The next night, more hallucinations followed by more prayers. This went on for weeks, I kept praying *asking God to guard my thoughts. "The peace of God, which transcends all understanding, will guard your hearts and your minds in Christ Jesus." Philippians 4:7 NIV*

Get To Peace

1. **Check In** – When was the last time you checked in with you? Anything holding you back? Are you anxious? Are you struggling physically, spiritually or mentally? Check in!

   Ask yourself, "How am I feeling?" Please share a few situations that currently concern you and open up. Also, share your feelings and what "resolution" would look like if you could solve the issue/change the situation.

2. **Therapy** – Resolving underlying or past issues is great for your health and peace of mind.

   Yes, seeking therapy to talk through issues is a great thing. There are times we are too close to an issue and need help to see things clearly. Fear may be the reason you're hesitant. What are you going to do in spite of the fear? Don't let fear win. Trust me, I understand if you are hesitant because, reaching out and admitting you have an issue is HUGE.

Take baby steps.

Step #1: Ask your doctor for a referral. Step #2: It may take interviewing a few counselors/doctors to find the right fit; look for your fit.

Step #3: Think about what is happening with you and be willing to share.

In preparation for your first therapy visit, what are three challenges you are facing?

3. **Self-Care** – Taking care of you should be your first priority. And, it is the only way you can be of service to others.

   What do you like to do for yourself that you've either given up or have been putting off? Think about it, and start doing it. Don't overthink it. Make time in your day or week for your self-care routine.

   Add one activity and continue to add on more until your heart is content. Recommendations: A facial, bubble bath, haircut, listening to music, reading or other hobbies. Be creative!

   What are five activities that you could try?

4. **Family Time** – Staying connected requires intention and preparation.

   Homes run smoothly when everyone participates and helps out. Everyone seems to be busy. The way to stay connected is to be prepared. Preparation can include pre-planning meals, assigning tasks for everyone each week, planning outside family meetings and outside activities, and scheduling for special events and projects.

   I recommend planning in advance for each week.

So what's your game plan this week? Please include at least three ways you can connect with your loved ones - be it quality time, working on projects or activities together or even having a weekly meal.

5. **Be Of Service** – We all have the ability to spread kindness wherever we find ourselves. Being of service can be in giving your time, your talents or your treasures.

    Serving could include: your church, your family, a group home, an organization in your community, or it could be a day of service event when you read to the children at the local library. Opportunities are everywhere.

    Where would you like to be of service?

    _____

    _____

    _____

6. **Finances** – I know this is another tough topic, but we must talk about budgeting, at least.

    My Dad talked to me about money and making sure I could stand on my own at all times. In his eyes, he never wanted his daughters to depend on a man - husband/boyfriend/friend.

    He would say, "Save for a rainy day." Basic budgeting is simply your earnings less expenses. In order to start budgeting, you must know where you stand. That means investing time in learning what you're spending, what you owe and what you are saving.

    Be truthful with yourself about all of your expenses:

    What are your earnings after taxes? (Weekly or monthly is fine)

How much do you owe monthly? (Mortgage/rent, utilities, telephone, insurance, subscriptions, etc.)

List them and then add them up.

How much do you spend weekly? (Groceries, gas, dining out, coffee shop visits, entertainment, etc.)

List them and add them up.

What is the balance of all your debt? (Include your credit cards, loans, and other debt)

Add it all.

Subtract the expenses from your earnings.

What is your remaining balance or loss?

Answering these questions will put you on the path to a healthier financial outlook because you know where you stand, and you'll be empowered to adjust where necessary.

If you need help creating a budget, *Google*, on your lunch break. Find a basic budget worksheet or check out Dave Ramsey's *"7 Baby Steps"* for some guidance to get you started.

7. **Spirituality** – Provides Protection, Strength, Confidence and Peace of Mind through connection with your Higher Power.

    When fear shows up, we must connect to something greater than us to find protection and guidance. Faith is a daily practice, and must be exercised like muscles.

    Spirituality – Lean into it. Pray and connect to your Higher Power. Praying each morning brings peace. It also helps to stay in balance, and to be connected to the wisdom needed to have small victories daily.

- Where do you find peace?
- Do you read the Bible daily?
- Do you listen to inspirational music or messages?
- Do you recite affirmations?
- Do you find peace in nature?

Let it fill your cup. Creating the habit of reading, reciting and then repeating (prayer/scripture/affirmation) keeps you connected to your hopes, dreams and allows God to minister to your heart.

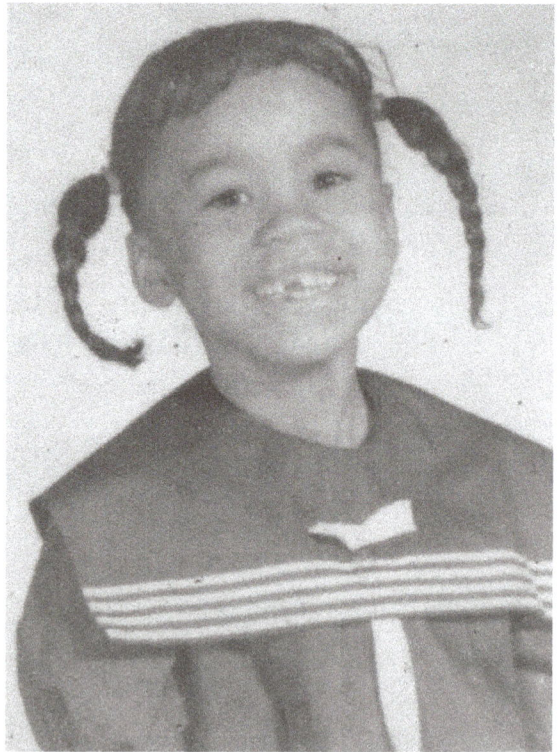

Little Lisa says, "Stay connected to your dreams."

Living My Best Life Play Lists

Enjoy every moment and every song in a no-judgment zone. Vibe out with the music.

Music has always been my go to; to calm my Spirit, to provide comfort when needed, and to dance - since I love dancing. During my recovery, I needed my music daily to keep my mood in check, and to stay motivated.

The mood I was in determined my Play List for the day. Some days I needed upbeat line dancing. There were days I needed to cry, and others when I needed be motivated, so I put on Gospel.

Each song helped me make it through that day's challenges. Perhaps you can enjoy them too!

Slide Songs And Line Dancing

Before I became paralyzed, I loved to dance and slide.
These are two of my favorites.

Cha Cha Slide, DJ Casper
Cupid Shuffle, Cupid

Why Me?

When I listened to these songs, they expressed my sadness, and what I couldn't say or admit out loud. They allowed me to connect with my pain and the sorrow of my condition.

Hear My Call, Jill Scott
Fill Me Up, Tasha Cobbs

My Smooth Jazz

When I was at peace and everything was going well, I found Smooth Jazz comforting and upbeat. On the weekends and after therapy when I could just relax, look out the window and enjoy, these songs kept me mellow.

Summer Rain, Jeanette Harris
Nightfall, Kim Waters
After The Storm, Norman Brown
The Way It Feels, Jeanette Harris

Inspirational Days

When I needed my Spirit lifted a little, these songs reminded me that God is in control. Even though I didn't understand all that was happening, I knew God was keeping me.

Your Spirit, Tasha Cobbs
Blessed & Highly Favored, The Clark Sisters
Open My Heart, Yolanda Adams
Major, Jekalyn Carr
Something Has To Break, Kierra Sheard

Victory

*Even though the odds are stacked against us at times,
never give up.*

*Keep fighting, keep pushing, keep grabbing and holding on
to every triumph God has given you!*

Go Get It, Mary Mary
Won't He Do It, Koryn Hawthorne
Walking, Mary Mary
Victory, Yolanda Adams

Lisa 2.0 - Dancing

*Get your groove on!
Go on out there, have some fun and enjoy each and
every step...
'cause none of them are promised.*

The Cookout, Cupid
Can't Get Enough, Tamia
Boots on the Ground, 803Fresh

Resources For Veterans

It's ok not to be ok and to need help working through any traumatic event. If you've experienced ANY abuse, seek help. Find a counselor, therapist or doctor, and talk it out.

For the Veteran's Crisis Line, dial 988 then press 1 or chat via text message to 838255.

To check your VA eligibility, please call 877-827-3702

The PVA (Paralyzed Veterans of America) is a great resource for navigating claims and benefits. They can be reached at 1-800-424-8200.

The St. Louis Region has a good reputation for supporting Veterans. The VA St. Louis Healthcare System and the VA Women's Clinic have contributed greatly to my recovery and healing. They can be contacted at:

VA St. Louis Healthcare System

VA.gov/st-louis-health-care
Main phone: 314-652-4100
VA Health connect: 833-381-1943
VA Mental Health care: 314-652-4100, ext. 66653
VA Women's Clinic VA.gov/st-louis-health-care/health-services/women-veteran-care

If you are not in St. Louis, there are facilities and clinics around the country. VA.gov/health

MyVA411 main information line   800-698-2411   Hours: 24/7

VA Benefits Hotline   800-827-1000

GI Bill Hotline   888-442-4551

National Call Center for   877-424-3838
Homeless Veterans

VA Health Benefits Hotline   877-222-8387

My Health Vet Help Desk   877-327-0022

A Note From The Publisher

Mission Possible Press...
Creating Legacies through Absolute Good Works

As a publisher, I have the opportunity to transform hopeful writers into successful authors. This brings me great pleasure because I believe everyone has wisdom to share and valuable stories to tell.

Being a caring person while facing some of the most difficult circumstances daily takes strength, courage and character. Sharing deep pain while being open and optimistic takes a calling, one I know Lisa Cooksey-Cannon is answering. Lisa shows us how to be our best selves during the most difficult times.

Thanks to Lisa Cooksey-Cannon, we are continuing to make the *Mission Possible-creating legacies, inspiring and building up - especially for families.* I am honored and pleased to present this book, *Victorious, A Journey Of Hope And Perseverance,* as part of our Extraordinary Living Series.

In the Spirit of Communication,

Jo Lena Johnson, Founder and Publisher
Mission Possible Press, a division of Absolute Good
AbsoluteGoodEnterprises.com

Acknowledgements

Lord, thank you for your grace, mercy, strength and guidance. You get all the glory. It has been the fight of my life; yet I made it through.

My Love, my soulmate, my husband and best friend. Thank you for holding my hand during this journey. Thank you for praying with and for me daily. Your support and care means everything.

My Sweetness, my beautiful daughter. The way you cared for me, loved on me, the way you prayed and researched every detail of my recovery was just amazing. Seeing your smile everyday gave me strength to keep pushing. Small victories daily is just the mantra I needed.

My Confidant, my loving sister. Thank you for coming and checking on me. I needed your calming spirit. Thank you for supporting each of us throughout this journey.

Thank you to my John Cochran ICU and Neurology teams, Dr. Caragine, Dr. Do, April, John, Alex, Mark, Nicole and Crystal. You answered all of our questions and extended grace when we needed things explained again and again. Your care allowed me to heal. God worked through your hands. I'm so thankful.

Thanks is not a big enough statement to express my gratitude to you, my Jefferson Barracks team. Each of you truly holds a special place in my heart. Lakeitha, Moe, Brenda, Carla, Maria, Shannon,

Val, Lyn, Amy, Kim, Matt, Charlie, Kat, Lars, Jackie, RaShonda, Dr. Krull, Dr. McCarthy, Nurse Laura and art therapist Laura, each of you played a huge part in my recovery. If I've missed a name or two, please forgive me. And, believe me when I say, your face and kindness will forever be written on my heart.

My church family, Church of the Living God, Temple of Faith, thank you for your prayers.

Doreen, Robin and Niecy, my squad. Thank you for your frequent visits and continuous prayers. Your obedience to God's Word helped me to get through each day. Our talks meant the world to me and your smiles brightened my days and my heart.

My classmates, neighbors and co-workers, thoughtful friends. Thank you for the visits, calls, baskets and flowers. Each token of kindness brightened my days. Carmen, J. Ross, Gordon, Donna, Haylee, Natalia & Daryl, Cheryl, Doris, Randy & Sara, Paul & Diane, Florence, Wendy, Marsha, Earl, Jacquie, John, Katie, Marty, Tracey, Michael & Jeanette, Sheldon, Quinton & JoAnn, Andy, Eboni, Kathy, Robert & Debbie.

And, thank you to the Paralyzed Veterans of America (PVA) for your support and assistance with navigating my health journey, benefits and the Veterans Administration process. Your organization, and Rodney, my Senior Benefits Advocate, make me proud, humbled and honored to be a Veteran of the United States Army.

About The Author

Lisa Cooksey-Cannon is a woman seeking God's heart. She's a Mom, wife, sister, aunt, step mother and grandmother. She grew up in the St. Louis, Missouri area and currently resides in Granite City, Illinois. She attended University City Senior High School. After graduation, she attended Southeast Missouri State University (SEMO) in Cape Girardeau, in pursuit of a teaching degree.

After a couple of years at SEMO, she decided to join the U.S. Army. She served 10 years in the army both on active duty, and served in the Reserves as well. She was stationed in Kaiserslautern, Germany, Colorado, California and Texas as a 71L, Administrative Specialist.

Lisa spent 30+ years working in the accounting field. She's held numerous positions in the accounting world: AP/AR, fixed assets, staff accountant, senior accountant, payroll manager and accounting manager. She's always willing to provide tips about accounting, personal finances and budgeting.

She loves to volunteer/community outreach. In the past, she's volunteered with Habitat for Humanity, St. Louis Area Foodbank, United Way of San Antonio and Boysville, Inc. She also participated in Toastmasters International where she held various club and district positions: Club President, Area Governor and District Treasurer. She retired… again in 2024 after her spinal cord injury. She loves reading a good book, journaling, completing puzzles, line dancing, attending live concerts and traveling.

www.ingramcontent.com/pod-product-compliance
Lightning Source LLC
Chambersburg PA
CBHW051534120626
46551CB00012B/1215